hospice

journey home

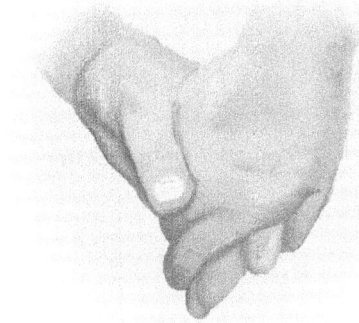

kim brandell

This is a work of fiction. No one depicted herein is real.

ISBN 978-0-9833987-8-3

Printed in the U.S.A. by
Smith Printing, LLC
Ramsey, MN 55303
(800) 416-9099 • www.smithprinting.com

For those who are young,
young at heart,
or those who are happily old
and understand that
someday, it'll be over.
If we can smile when we die,
it is a testament to the rich
and happy life we've lived.

Smile.

table of contents

chapter

one

When he was born in 1940, the world, the entire world, was his to explore. He could go damn near anywhere. In 1942, he traveled to St. Paul in a car, without a car-seat or seat-belt, in the roomy compartment of an old Chevy, with two smokers, yellowed upholstery and dark, poisonous air; and in 1965, he travelled to Da Nang, South Vietnam on a jet, with three aisles, ashtrays filled with spent cigarettes and 365 nervous soldiers squirming in seats constructed for people half their size. From ages two to twenty-five, from St. Paul to Da Nang, he could go damn near anywhere. In 1969, when a spacecraft landed on the Moon and a man with moon dirt under his feet said *One giant leap for mankind*, his world expanded beyond earth. It was possible. He could go further. He could travel to Africa, Australia, Lithuania, Topeka, the Philippines, the Yucatan, Vietnam, Point Barrow or the Moon. Man had been there; he could go. Money, time and technology were necessary, but it was plausible, within the realm of possibility. Anywhere. Damn near anywhere. As a younger man, he closed his eyes and dreamed. *I can go damn near anywhere. Wow!*

On August 8, 2015, the 75 year old was wheeled into his bedroom. The chair, a *Midline,* manufactured in New York and labeled **Mercy Hospital Oncology**, had been busy. Thirty-two sick and dying patients had rested on its leather seat in the two days before he was gently moved from a hospital bed to a wheelchair, for the trip home. The leather arm rests were worn and cracked, the gaps filling with the dead skin of cancer patients who had lost hope. Old, but functional, the *Midline*, carrying another sick and dying patient, crossed the threshold without sound, without power, except that generated by the man who held the handles and pushed, and delivered him home.

Strapped in the chair, slouching, stretching the straps and creasing his old, leathery skin, he was rolled into his old home, his new home, his hospice. One man, a black man, pushed the chair while another, a white man, opened the door and cleared the way. They were large men, much larger than him. They were strong, prominent, beefy; he was frail, disappearing and weak. Both men were dressed in white, both spoke softly and each wore a sympathetic smile, permanently imprinted on their faces by their job. The black man had worked for Allina Hospice since 2000 and the white man since 1985. Both had responded to an ad placed in the *Classifieds* of *The Minneapolis Tribune,* written with the same words in 1985 as in 2000. Some things never change. *Transport terminal patients, by motor vehicle and wheelchair from hospital to hospice. Competitive salary and benefits available. Compassion and a drivers' license required.*

He opened his tired eyes. His bedroom had changed. It was almost unrecognizable. While he was gone, while he received treatment and lost hope, it had changed. Warmth had been replaced by sterility, and familiarity and comfort, gave way to plastic bins filled with rubber tubes, rubber gloves and boxes of *Adult Pampers*. His *Tempur-Pedic* was gone, and in its place, moored to the carpet by gravity and legs on wheels, sat an adjustable bed, with side-rails made of cream-colored, rounded plastic poles. The side-rails were designed to keep the sick in bed. He was sick; the side-rails were designed to keep him in bed. The side-rail furthest from the door was up and locked, and the one closest to the door, was down, giving the men in white easy access to the bed when moving him from his chair and converting him from mobile to bedridden and dying.

When the *Midline* was adjacent to the bed, after its wheels stopped turning and it was locked in place, one man, the black man, lifted him by his armpits, while the other elevated his old, flat ass from the chair. It took little strength to lift him, he weighed now what he weighed when he was twelve, 108-pounds. They boosted him out of the chair, separating his elbows from the arm rests, leaving his dead skin on the chair's arms, to be eaten by cracks in the leather and to join the dead skin of those who preceded him. As he hovered above the chair, the man who held him by his arm pits, unlocked the chair with his left foot, moved the chair out of the way with his right foot, and then both men in white and their cargo, 108 pounds of disease and despair, moved to the side, where the men in white softy laid him in the bed. A man in white, lifted the lowered bedrail and locked it in place. *To keep the sick in bed.*

The other man in white, the African-American who had hair only on the sides of his head, pushed a button and the back third of the bed rose in the direction of the overhead light. When the back of the bed rose 45-degrees, he lifted his finger from the button and the bed's ascent ended. He wedged a pillow between the mattress and bedridden man's back, handed him the button, backed away five feet, so he could better inspect his work, smiled, satisfied he was comfortable and secure, and asked him, "How's that?"

It was fine. It was what he expected, consistent with history. He had been in this position plenty before and knew what to expect. They had done what was expected. There were limitations. He knew that, but he also knew that neither of the men could do anything about the limitations. "It's fine, thank you."

"Anything else we can do? We're here. We can do what you want."

They couldn't do anything about the limitations. They couldn't change what was unchangeable. It was inevitable. Radiation hadn't changed it, nor had surgery or chemotherapy. Inevitable. Preordained? Maybe, but either way, nothing could change it. "No. Thanks for all you've done. I appreciate it."

The black man in white took hold of a small and shrinking right hand, a hand as much of swollen veins as flesh and bone, and held it for a long two seconds. With words and sympathetic eyes, he said goodbye. "Mr. Thomas, it has been a pleasure to know you. I wish you the best."

The best? There is no best. It's all inevitable. Obdurate. It's over. "Thank you. You have done a *yeoman's job* and I appreciate it."

As the man in white turned to leave the room, as he began to close the door behind him, Mr. Thomas called out to him. His voice was weak, but his words were strong. "If you need a refer-ence, let me know, but you better ask soon."

The Black man, the man in white, the one who helped lift Mr. Thomas to his hospital bed with side-rails, the one who wished him his best, heard Mr. Thomas' pledge of support, turned, smiled broadly, saluted the son of a sailor, the son of *Old Sea Dad*, and left the room.

Mr. Thomas smiled. *A yeoman's job. Old Sea Dad* knew and he had told his son, Paul Thomas. *Old Sea Dad* had learned of yeomen while on a ship, on his way to Okinawa. Yeomen completed the Navy's paperwork and they got it right, because they had to. No choice. Mistake free. Errors in Navy paper-work empowered the Japanese. They got it right. America won *Old Sea Dad's* War. "*A yeoman's job*, is a job well done," he called out, but because his voice was weak and the nearly bald black man was likely near the front door, out of range, he didn't hear. "A yeoman's job. Thank you."

When the door closed, he was alone. No doctors who looked at charts, scans and biopsy results that provided no hope, and no nurses who adjusted bags that hung from a pole and asked ques-tions that had no answers. He was alone.

The doctor told him to go home, that nothing more could be done. He told him to go home and live the remainder of his life in peace. *Die at home.* Without more acceptable options, he said, *Okay.*

Not the Yucatan, not Point Barrow, not Lithuania, not even St. Paul. The moon still circled his world, men still dreamed of leaving tracks in moon dirt, but his dreams no longer included lift-off and a lunar landing. His world was now his room, a large sterile corner in a comfortable home in Minnesota. As an old and sick man, he closed his eyes and dreamed, but the realistic possibilities were limited. There was then and now and only here. His room.

Safe, secure, unable to fall from his bed, locked in, he closed his eyes and slept.

chapter
two

Paul Thomas had Stage IV lung cancer. He started smoking at 12, before anyone knew it was dangerous, when everyone believed it was cool, daring, mature and attractive. When he first heard rumbles that cigarettes were not good for his health, he was 16 and smoking a pack a day. By the time he graduated from law school, the Surgeon General had determined that cigarettes caused cancer and he was smoking two and a-half packs of cigarettes a day. While trudging through swamps and tall grass, trying to avoid North Vietnamese booby traps, a smoke relaxed him, and given the environment, relaxation was more important than good health. When discharged and home, he was nearly thirty-years old, and published, credible studies concluded, smoking led to cancer, heart disease and other crippling maladies, but by then he had been smoking nearly two-thirds of his life and in spite of his best efforts, he was unable to quit.

He attended classes sponsored by the American Lung Association, designed to help people kick the tobacco habit, and when the class ended, he was smoke-free for nearly a day. He submitted to hypnosis and was given a post-hypnotic suggestion designed to kill the craving, but smoked in the car on the way home from his session. Acupuncture didn't help and when he filled a prescription for Nicorette, a gum that was to satisfy cravings for nicotine while the cigarette habit was kicked, he discovered Nicorette was best when chewed, while smoking a Camel.

In 1952, at 12, he drew in the smoke from a cigarette he had found smoldering on the sidewalk, and on June 10, 2013, 61-years later, the doctor ordered an x-ray, and after consulting with a radiologist and oncologist, told him, "Mr. Thomas, I'm afraid you have lung cancer."

"How bad is it?"

"I can't say; I'm not an oncologist, but the mass is large. I've made an appointment for you at an oncologist's office in Coon Rapids for Thursday. With your permission, I'll send him my records. He'll have better or more complete answers than I have."

"You have my permission."

"Are you a smoker, Mr. Thomas?"

"Yes I am. Started young and haven't kicked the habit."

"How much do you smoke?"

He had cut down to 35 cigarettes a day. "A little less than a pack a day." It was a fib, a bend of the truth. *Why lie? It won't shrink the mass or contribute to the efficacy of treatment. Why say 15 when it's really 35?* He didn't know why he lied, but he had, and even though he was given an opportunity to set the record straight, to tell the truth, to confess his dishonesty, while the Doctor made notes in his file, he didn't. In fact, he doubled down and confirmed what wasn't true. "Yeah, just under a pack a day."

"Well, as you know, smoking isn't good for your health. I'd suggest you stop. You have a battle on your hands, and you'll be better suited for battle if the cigarettes aren't part of your armor."

Paul knew he was right, had known it since he was 16 years old, since 1956, when young World War II veterans were recent college graduates and the United States was emerging as the big kid on the World's block. The message wasn't new, it had resonated for years. *Quit. Quit. Quit.*

After signing release forms so his old doctor could send his new doctor private and confidential information, Paul walked to his car. He parked it at the far end of the clinic's parking lot, so he would be required to walk a long way, to exercise his heart and lungs. *What for? Why? A lot of good it did me. Bull shit.*

He climbed in his car, behind the wheel, lit a cigarette and cried. Although the answer was clear, through tears he asked, *Why me?*

When he arrived home to his house on the river, the home where he raised three children and six dogs, he parked in his stall and walked into the kitchen. He was reluctant to tell his wife what the doctor had found. Every day for 45 years, she told him to quit or die. He listened, he tried, but didn't do as she pleaded with him to do. She was right. She had every right to tell him, *I told you so.* He didn't want to hear it. He'd heard enough for one day.

She looked away from the dinner she was preparing, brushed a blonde curl from her flour covered forehead and asked, "Well?"

"Not a cold."

"Flu?"

"Nope."

"What then?"

"Lung cancer."

Gently, she rested utensils in bowls and walked to him. As tears filled her eyes, she took him in her arms, held him close and whispered, "We'll get through this. One way or the other, we'll get through this together."

In the two years following his diagnosis, although Paul continued to smoke consistent with his lie, 15 cigarettes a day, a reduction occasioned by his ill-health or his unwillingness to live a lie, Mary never said, *I told you so*. She stood by him, drove him when he couldn't, cleaned his vomit after chemo-therapy, nursed his wounds after surgery, fed him and propped up his spirits when treatment and impending doom brought him down, but never said, *I told you so*.

Paul was unlucky in health, lucky in love. Mary was an angel constructed of tempered, rust-proofed steel. Her strength was forged as a child, fortified as a young woman and employed when Paul needed it most.

Mary's dad died when she was six, of alcohol poisoning and her mom tried to quickly follow his suit by drinking until drunk every day from his death, until she was committed as chemically dependent and mentally ill, 18 years later. After a trial, the judge committed her to a state-owned treatment facility, where she died at 45.

Paul was Mary's mother's court-appointed attorney. Mary had cooperated with the County in its attempts to commit her mother, believing it was best for her to stop drinking and that she could not do it on her own. She signed the Petition which asked a judge to send her to treatment and provided testimony in court, as a witness for the County. The first words Paul ever spoke to her, were in the courtroom.

"Is it really your wish that your mother, the woman who gave birth to you, be locked in a facility with mentally ill and chemically dependent people?"

"It's my wish that my mother get better."

"And do you think she'll get better in a state hospital?"

"I'm not sure."

"You're not sure and yet you're asking the Court to commit her to a locked facility a hundred-miles from her home?"

"Yes."

"Then pray tell, why?"

"Because nothing else has worked. My dad died 18 years ago, and she has been drowning her sorrow in alcohol ever since. If she doesn't get help soon, she'll die."

The questioning continued. Although Paul attempted to compromise Mary's opinion by asking her about alternatives to court-ordered involuntary treatment, she was intractable. Small, fit, sitting straight in the witness chair, brushing blonde curls from her blue eyes and speaking clearly, slowly, Mary never wavered. She told Paul and the Court that she had tried everything, all of the options that were suggested by Paul as lesser restrictive alternatives to mandated treatment, and that her mother rejected them or tried them and failed. Her opinion was firm, her testimony resolute.

A doctor offered testimony that supported the County's request and the County rested its case. Paul called no witnesses. He could find no doctor to support the suggestion that Mary's mother be released, and Mary was her mother's only child and no other friend or member of extended family was willing to testify in support of her release. Paul considered asking her to testify, but after a consultation with her, a meeting that revealed she was obstinate, irrational, chemically dependent and mentally-ill, he decided against it.

The judge committed Mary's mother as mentally-ill and chemically dependent. She received court-ordered professional help at a state-owned hospital in northwestern Minnesota and three-months after she arrived, she died.

A month after Paul learned that his client and Mary's Mother had died, Mary made an appointment to meet with him. She sat across the desk from Paul, wearing the same blue dress and beige sweater she wore in court, and pleaded her case. "I was right. Even though my mother died in that hospital, I was right."

Paul said nothing. He digested what had been said and visually inspected the woman who appeared before him. She was pleasant looking, mid-twenties, blonde, appropriately dressed, relatively fit and broken. There was something askew, something not quite right. Although Paul suspected the quirk may have been a consequence of her mother's recent death and her participation in the process that may have contributed to her early demise, he thought it went beyond that.

"When you questioned me, you seemed to suggest I was doing something wrong, that I didn't love my mother. That's not true. I loved her and wanted what was best for her and I thought commitment was her only answer."

"And maybe it was. I'm sorry your mother died. I don't hold you responsible. I believe you said what you thought was right. Your mother didn't die because you testified in Court, she died for the reasons that brought you there. Your mom was sick. You saw that and simply asked the Court to see it as well."

Mary said nothing. She grieved her mother's death and grieved her participation in that death. *If I hadn't testified, if I hadn't signed the Petition, if she had stayed home and continued to drink, if I hadn't interfered, would she be here? Would she have survived? Would she have found help her way?* Paul had exonerated her, explained that she was right, that she did the right thing, but she had not yet forgiven herself. She sat in a chair in a lawyer's office and wept.

"I'm sorry if I made it harder. I didn't mean to. My job was to challenge the County's position and that meant cross-examining you. I'm sorry. I know you loved your mother and did what you could do."

Like a Jack-in–the-Box with a broken spring, a door with a faulty hinge or a 1932 Packard with a flat tire, Mary wiped tears from her eyes, looked at her mother's lawyer and reluctantly and clumsily accepted his apology. "Thank you, it's hard."

Paul took Mary to lunch. He discovered she was alone, separated from two parents by liquor. She had no siblings, few close friends and lived in the basement of the church where her Mother's funeral had been. She was broken, abandoned, a disillusioned woman in need of rescue. And rescue her he did.

After they abandoned the hauntings of their history, they dated. Paul discovered Mary was broken, but not irreparable. She needed love, consistency and patience, to combat her years of isolation, years when she mothered her mother and tried to do what could not be done. With a little help from Paul, Mary fixed herself. She emerged from the year anniversary of her mother's death, happy, secure, optimistic, independent and in love.

In 1968, Paul and Mary said, *I do*. Forty-seven years later, 49 years after Paul tried to dry Mary's tears with an explanation, Mary tried to dry Paul's with a hug.

He woke, leaning against the bedrail. Thank God for the bedrail. Without it, he would have fallen to the floor. *To keep the sick in bed.*

Mary was at his bedside, fidgeting with her iPad. She had always taken to new technology quicker than Paul.

When dot-matrix printers were the rage, she purchased one, and by intuition or by instructions, four minutes after it was rescued from a box, she inserted an ink cartridge, fed paper through its cover, hit a button and it printed a page of numbers in 100-seconds. When Paul was trying to determine how to open his newly purchased flip-phone, Mary was texting their kids with hers. She abandoned internet by telephone, the day broadband became available in their neighborhood and purchased a wireless modem and went wireless while all of her friends were still waiting for the phone line to clear. She had three email addresses, one for family, one for friends and one for commercial contacts, and was able to integrate them so she could receive messages as they were sent, as she wanted them. She corrected erroneous entries on Wikipedia and used four search engines to gather uncontroverted information.

She used AOL Chat, left it for My Space and landed on Facebook. She had 376 followers and posted at least three times daily. When her kids couldn't figure it out, they called Mom. When computers and smart-phones went off-kilter, when smart-phones lost their intelligence or their printers wouldn't print, they didn't ask their kids, they called Mom, and invariably, she fixed the problem.

"Trump says he's really rich and most Mexicans who cross the border are rapists and murderers. Asshole."

Mary formulated her political views while working for a non-profit that provided shelter to homeless families. She had a masters' degree in social work when she applied to work for Anoka County Helps Impoverished Families (ACHIF). ACHIF had two positions available. One required a master's degree and the hired person was to develop programing designed to break the cycle of poverty. It was a paperwork job that required skill and paid well. Although Mary was qualified for the programing position, she didn't apply for it. Mary applied for and received a position identified in the ad, as *the Roundup*. According to the Help Wanted Ad that appeared in the *Minneapolis Tribune* in June, 1981, the *Roundup is responsible for, Greeting, Supervising and Serving ACHIF's Most Important People, the Families it Serves. The qualified candidate must have a high school diploma and be willing to work closely with people who are impoverished.*

Although management attempted to convince Mary to accept the programmer's position, she was hired as the *Roundup*. For nearly thirty years, Mary worked the floor of a deteriorating shelter in Columbia Heights, a first ring suburb, north of Minneapolis. Her clients became her friends. They struggled as her mom had struggled, often chemically dependent, mentally ill or like her mom, both. They gave birth to children, loved them and were unwilling to give them away, but didn't have the wherewithal to care for them. They asked the government for help and received it, but it wasn't enough. Most were unable to work, unable to earn enough money to feed and house their families, and many were not successful in working the system to obtain subsidized housing, food stamps and disability benefits. They asked the County for help, but funds were limited, workers scarce and lines for help long. They slipped between the cracks and found themselves on the doorstep of ACHIP. According to Mary, they were nice, loving, friendly, honest and kind, but in need of an advocate.

Mary often returned home from work, tired and frustrated. She often shouted *Why?*, without waiting for an answer. She screamed, she cursed, she cried, she tried to convince Paul to open their home to families unable to find a bed at the shelter. He said, *No.*

On cold nights, when temperatures dipped lower than twenty-five below, the shelter filled and Mary was required to turn away cold families and explain that they needed to find alternative shelter. She gave the rejected families business cards with telephone numbers and addresses where they could seek assistance, but she knew few would reach out and many would sleep in doorways or warm themselves by entering restaurants where they would remain until management determined they were not paying customers and escort them into the cold. Some would be rescued by police, others would suffer frostbite and spend the night in an emergency room or hospital. How resources were allocated never made sense to Mary.

"It costs more money to hospitalize a family after it suffers from exposure, than it costs us to house and feed 40 families for a night. Cops can't fight crime if they're finding a warm place for a cold family. It makes no sense."

Paul was sympathetic, but not as blindly compassionate as Mary. "A line needs to be drawn. If not, where will it end? I don't like practicing law, but I do, because I need money to care for my family. People need to make choices, and some of those choices aren't attractive."

"They have few choices. They're mentally ill, drunk or suffering from a transient setback that could end with some short-time assistance. They don't choose to be there. They have no choice."

"But, Social Security helps the disabled and Human Services provides cash public assistance, food stamps and subsidized housing. There is help and those who are unable to find it, need only call the County and someone paid by you and me, a public servant, will do everything humanly possible to keep them from the cold."

"But, it's not that easy. Language barriers, red tape, bureaucratic complexities, all make it hard. Some just give up."

"Maybe they shouldn't give up."

"Maybe they shouldn't, but they do, and when they do, they're cold and vulnerable and have no options."

"But they had options and chose to not take advantage of available services. I understand you want to help, and you are helping, but many of the problems they face are self-created. If there were more shelters, there would be more people using them. You turn people away with only one shelter in Anoka County. If we had three, you'd still turn people away. You can't fix it. I can't fix it and the government can't fix it."

Mary wiped a tear from the corner of her right eye. "But, they have so little and so many have so much. It's not fair."

Paul was not unsympathetic. He had dried Mary's tears on many cold nights, had shed a few himself and wished there was a solution. He'd pay his fair share. He would be happy to drive a compact rather than an SUV, if it meant there would be no homeless, hungry people. He would have worked a year beyond his targeted retirement age, if it meant most children could go to sleep each night with a warm blanket, soft bed and full stomach. He would sacrifice a meal at an expensive restaurant, tickets to the baseball game, an extra pair of shoes or the television in the basement, the TV that is turned on only three times a year, if he believed his sacrifices would alleviate hunger, pain and homelessness, but he didn't believe they would. "It's not fair, but neither is life. It's not a problem that can be solved by throwing money at it. It's cultural, it's genetic, it's complicated."

"Why should Carl drive a $150,000.00 car, while a family I couldn't find a bed for tonight, is forced to sleep in a doorway? For a hundred-dollars, they could be warm in a cheap motel. Maybe the money Carl spent on his car, should be used to buy motel rooms for the homeless families."

Paul understood what her heart had said. He got it. He didn't want people to be hungry and cold. He got it, but he also believed Carl had a right to his expensive car and that his pursuit of a Maserati, meant jobs for those he employed. But, that was economics and Mary was talking compassion. Sometimes they met, sometimes they didn't. Empathizing with his wife and sympathizing with cold children on the street, Paul kept economics in his pocket and peacefully surrendered. "Maybe you're right."

Donald Trump was not someone Mary admired. When he announced his candidacy, she laughed. When media coverage of his campaign dominated air waves, she became concerned and asked, "Can this jerk win?"

Paul didn't think so. He was not as liberal as Mary, but believed civility and experience were prerequisites to the presidency, so took Trump lightly. *No civility, no experience, no chance.* "No. Not a prayer."

"God, I hope not. What a jerk."

Mary put her iPad on the end of the bed with side-rails, made a few political statements and asked a question. "He's trying to inflame the rednecks with all this anti-Mexican talk. A wall. A joke. Him and his wall, both jokes. How'd you sleep?"

"Fine. Drugs do wonders."

After his diagnosis and failed treatments, Paul was in pain. His body hurt everywhere. His joints were inflexible and when forced to move, silently screamed in pain. His lungs ached or burned, depending on the day, and when he coughed, which was often, the pain intensified and radiated to his throat. He suffered daily from headaches, caused either by anti-cancer medicines or the presence of carcinogens that had migrated from his lungs to his cerebellum. When he ate, his stomach told him it was digesting barbed-wire, when he urinated, it burned like he was pissing acid, when he defecated, it hurt, suggesting he was passing razor-blades and when he stretched while sitting on the toilet, to reach down and wipe, his back creaked and asked him to stop. *Please Stop!*

When pain was mixed with impending doom, the emotional blackness that descended when he learned there was nothing more to do, that the end was near, Paul prayed the end come quickly. If it was simply a matter of time, he wanted the time to be short. *Get on with it. Be done. Let's go. Get on with it. Now!* He was unwilling to hasten his death by firearm, rope or carbon monoxide, afraid of the eternal consequences, but wanted it to end. *Soon! Now!*

He explained his wish for a hastened demise to his oncologist, who offered two, mutually exclusive, simple solutions. "We can stop the administration of all medicine, which will quicken the process, but you'll die in pain, or we can administer strong anti-pain medication which will alleviate pain and buoy your spirits and as a result, extend your life."

Paul chose the first option. He was ready. *I'm done. Get on with it!* He could no longer sire children, embark on a journey to St. Paul or the moon, or change the world. There wasn't much left, just pain and the interminable wait. He envied those who died of a massive heart attack or stroke. He wished he could have been so lucky. "Nope. No drugs. Let's do this fast. But thanks for the options Doc."

Three days later, he changed his mind. He was an old, dying, stiff, but was capable of transformation, a metamorphosis. He chose a different option.

His daughter, Lauren, 45, the divorced mother of two college-aged children, a girl and a boy, came to visit him in the hospital. She was lovely, warm and pretty, bright and upbeat. She remembered tennis with Paul. He taught her when she was five-years old and she became a better player than him before she reached high school. They spent hours at the courts, father and daughter, tennis racquets and balls. As she shared her recollections with her father, the cancer patient who had decided a rush to death was the best option, she smiled, returning to a simpler time, a time when there was time. A time when the future was theirs, and their futures were bright. She tried to resurrect the happiness they shared when younger, with a sentimental trip to another, earlier day, a day when the sun shined, the clouds were puffy and white and the wind, a welcomed light breeze that cooled father and daughter, but Paul's diagnosis and resistance shrouded him in sadness and pain. Because he was consumed by death and pain, and unwilling to reach for comfort, Paul didn't remember, he didn't smile, but instead battled pain in his hands, his chest, his feet and his head.

Lauren stood to leave, kissed her coach and father on the forehead, smiled and said, "See you tomorrow." Before walking from the room, Lauren paused, turned and looked again at her father. She was 45 and 5 at the same time, young Lauren and older Lauren, the future and a memory from the past. As her eyes filled with tears, she smiled. She silently begged her father for more, a chance, an opportunity to say goodbye while reveling in their shared and beautiful past. Her pause was a plea, an overture, a silently articulated question, an invitation to explore and remember.

As she stood before him, without words, pleading for opportunities, Paul determined the wait, previously thought of as interminable and painful, gave him time to remember, explore, smile and say, *I love you.* He concluded there was a better way to die, a way that would allow him to share in the joys his life had created.

Hospice. Paul knew hospice. He'd been there before. He hadn't died, hadn't been a hospice patient, but he'd been there before. He knew hospice.

After his mother died, Paul volunteered to provide hospice care to terminally ill patients. His mother was surrounded by family when she died, given a warm goodbye by those she loved and for whom she cared. She was at peace when she slipped away, in the spiritual arms of her friends, son, daughter-in-law and grand-children and was able to breathe her last breath only minutes af-ter being hugged and kissed. As her life ended, it was clear to her that it had a purpose, clear that it left an appreciative, walking, talking, breathing legacy.

A peaceful passage surrounded by loved ones, was a luxury Paul knew others didn't have. He knew people died alone, forgotten. He surmised, they passed anxious, without comfort or validation. He wanted to provide comfort, and warmth, a peaceful presence, to the extent he could, and volunteered to care for terminally ill patients in need of conversation, warmth and friendship, a nice guide to the hereafter.

After a ten-minute meeting with a hospice nurse, during which he learned the key to hospice care was presence, Paul was asked to provide eleventh-hour care for a woman near death. She laid on her back, in a bed, in a nursing home that cared for 63 dying patients.

The old woman's head was large, her body small, her hair short and wispy, her complexion, gray. Paul sat at her bedside, stifling a cigarette smoker's cough and watched her mouth open to take in air and close, to keep moisture in. Paul wasn't sure. He didn't know what to do. If he spoke, would she hear? If she heard, would she welcome his kind but clumsy words, or bristle at the stranger's attempt to disturb her peaceful rest? If she woke and lifted her large head from the pillow and tried to stand, would he help her find the floor or discourage the attempt, and if he did and she resisted, what would he do? Get physical with a dying, 92 year old woman who weighed as much as Paul's left leg?

But, she didn't wake. An hour after Paul arrived, a squatty nurse in white, entered the room and raised the head of the bed, without siderails. Startled, the old woman opened her eyes, and without shifting her head, scanned the room with darting eyes. The nurse gently pinched the old woman's cheeks and when her lips parted, dropped two pills in her mouth. As the nurse tipped a glass of cold water to the old woman's parched mouth, the terminally-ill nonagenarian took hold of the glass and helped the nurse pour water into her mouth and flush the pills to their intended destination. When the old woman quenched her thirst, and washed medicine down her throat, she and the nurse, both holding the glass partially filled with water, tipped the glass so that it was upright and resting on an elderly chest. The nurse attempted to take the glass from the old woman, but her ancient grip was surprisingly tight and the nurse abandoned her effort, leaving the tall glass with water, in the old woman's cupped hands, resting on her chest.

Alone with the dying cancer patient, Paul watched the water-filled glass rise and fall each time the old woman inhaled and exhaled. When she twitched or coughed, the glass tilted and water reached the edges of its captivity and threatened to spill onto the old woman's pajamas. Twice Paul reached for the glass and tried to gently pull it from its captor, but each time he did, the old woman tightened her grip, opened her eyes and scowled at Paul.

For three hours, Paul was not concerned about the old woman's comfort, her breathing, her potential last breath or passage to the next place, he was focused on the glass and the water that threatened peace. He tried to forget, attempted to ignore the waves created by breathing and coughing, but could not. He watched, and watched and watched. The glass, the water, the waves, her grip on the glass and life, was his focus, his rumination.

When his relief appeared, Paul told her the old woman was resting comfortably and that her breathing was shallow and regular, and when he stood and pulled his jacket on, watched the replacement volunteer, take hold of the glass and when the older woman resisted, heard her say, *That's okay Grace, I'm just taking the glass so you don't spill.* As she sat Paul's muse on a table and averted a wet disaster, she smiled and added, *Thanks Paul, I'm sure Grace appreciates your presence.*

Paul knew hospice, an opportunity for peace, reflection, painless passage.

"Dad, I said I'll see you tomorrow." Lauren smiled at her father who laid in a bed fortified with side-rails; Paul did not smile, but wanted to. The pain and the impending doom precluded him from enjoying reflections on his life, the 75-years before cancer, before pain, the 75-years of sharing, loving, contributing and living. He wanted to smile, to accept her invitation, to return to the good days, to re-live a life lived fully and happily. He wanted to share joy with those he loved, while he could. *Get on with it? Fast? Sprint to the grave? Foreclose opportunities? Wrong answer. Bullshit.*

Paul accepted Lauren's invitation to relive happiness while on his way to another place. He was transformed, a butterfly, once a caterpillar, a child, once a prayer, a man who wanted to live, once a man who wanted to die. He pushed the button used to call a nurse, and when she arrived, he asked to talk to his doctor. Later that evening the doctor stood at the end of Paul's bed and received new instructions. The butterfly, prayer and man who wanted to live, said, "Give me whatever there is to relieve the pain and lift my spirits. I know I'm going to die, but I want to do it with a smile on my face."

Ten minutes later, a nurse injected him with a concoction, and five minutes thereafter, the pain magically disappeared. Not only did the pain dissolve, his spirits were lifted. He wasn't delusional; he didn't think he'd beat the cancer and return to the tennis court with his daughter. He knew he'd soon die, but, in the meantime, he'd live pain free, immersed in memories of a life well lived. They'd return to the courts while he laid in bed. With a glass of cold water on the table beside him, he called Lauren and asked, *What time tomorrow?*

A month later, in his bedroom, where he was and where he would be until he was no more, laying in a bed with side-rails, a bed that stood on wheels and lifted his head when he told it to do so with his finger on a button, the drugs still worked. They hadn't cured his cancer; they hadn't stalled its progress, but it had given him the opportunity to live his final days with a smile on his face, a smile spawned by family, friends and memories. Paul looked at his wife of 40-years, the mother of his children, the person with whom he shared his most important and joyful moments, the person with whom he shared his most painful and insignificant moments, and accepting her political passions and understanding she wanted her dying husband to be an ally, not a combatant, said, "Yeah, he's a prick. A wall? My ass."

chapter three

*M*ary handed Paul two remote controls, one to turn on the television and another to change the television's channels. "There you go. Just like at the hospital. Everything at your fingertips."

"At the hospital, when I tried to change channels, I raised my bed and when I tried to turn off the television, I called the nurse." Paul's inability to determine which was which, plagued him and the nurses station. When the news was over, he tried to turn off the television, to sleep in relative quiet, and in spite of his button pushing, the set remained on, while a nurse entered the room, out-of-breath and red faced, asking, *Is anything wrong?* When Paul tired of *The View* and wanted *Jeopardy*, he pushed, but *The View* remained on-screen and another exasperated nurse appeared in the doorway.

Eventually, the charge nurse took charge of the television remote control and asked Paul to push the only button she left for him, the *Call Nurse* button, when he wanted to change channels, and she'd respond and come to his room and change the television channel. Her plan worked, but there was a delay. A remote control was immediate, a summoned nurse, not so. Nurses didn't always promptly respond to Paul's calls. When a nurse saw a light flashing, summoning her to Paul's room, she assumed it wasn't urgent, but rather a request to act as a channel changer. Sometimes, she was with another cancer patient, administering life-saving, pain-taking measures, and couldn't leave a needy patient to change *American Idol* to *Eyewitness News*. Paul depressed the button, waited and fumed. Paul began anticipating the delay and pushed the button at 9:45, for a change he wanted at 10:00.

It became all too routine. Whenever Paul pushed the *Call Nurse* button, a nurse looked, saw it was Paul calling, concluded it was like all other calls he placed, a request to change a channel and responded only when convenient. Twenty days after Paul was admitted to the hospital, four days after the protocol designed to limit the inconvenience caused by Paul's inability to distinguish between the remote control and *Call Nurse* button was implemented, the incision from Paul's surgery began oozing. The mix of blood and puss flowed from the banks of his wound and escaped the gauze dam, and began to crawl along his stomach and fall to the bed. There were no visitors in his room, so Paul pushed the *Call Nurse* button. He waited and waited, while the ooze pooled on the bed, ruined his sheets and soiled his butt. When the nurse finally responded to the call, 35 minutes after it was placed, she looked at Paul, held the television's remote control in hand and said, "Channel?"

The protocol was scrapped, the wound was cleaned and the bedsheets discarded and replaced.

As Paul was about to remind Mary of remotes and the complications they create, he began to cough. And cough and cough. His lungs were trying to expel carcinogens through his mouth. It didn't work, but they tried, over and over and over. He coughed until his throat burned and his lungs ached. Little was expelled, save sour air, but the coughing went on and on. When the fit finally ended, Paul was exhausted and the tale he was to tell, forgotten.

Mary offered her dying husband cold water and wiped expectorant from his chin and the corners of his mouth. She dropped the soiled tissue into the garbage can where it joined others.

Weakly, Paul shooed his helper from the room. "That took it out of me. I'm tired. I'm going to sleep. Thanks for being here."

"I wouldn't be anywhere else. Need anything before I go?"

"No. I just need sleep."

Mary left the bedroom, leaving the door open a crack, so she could monitor her husband without opening the sticky and potentially noisy door. She clutched her iPad with her right hand, waved *Goodbye* with her left, smiled and walked out of Paul's hospice and into the living room of their home on the river.

Paul closed his eyes. *Not fun. Dying isn't what it's cracked up to be. Shit.* Before he could add another derisive comment to his personal condemnation of death, he was asleep.

Two hours after he fell asleep, after imaginary bouts with large women in tights and small men in tuxedos, Paul woke and when he opened his eyes, he saw Lauren standing over him. "Do you remember Sunday mornings in the summer, at the courts?"

There was no *Hello,* no *Welcome back.* There would have been; Lauren wouldn't have launched into conversation without a greeting, so Paul concluded that there had been, that after greetings were exchanged, he had fallen asleep again and he had forgotten. He rejoined the conversation midstream, believing cancer had interrupted again. "I remember."

"You were so patient. I couldn't hit the ball, but you kept tossing them my way. When I finally did hit one over the net, you acted as if we'd landed on the Moon. You made such a big deal out of my lucky hit. You were so proud. You made me proud of myself. It worked. Your enthusiasm became mine and I fell in love with tennis. Sunday mornings. We skipped church, but worshipped in our own, special way on Sunday mornings."

"We did. I remember." He did and the memory made him smile.

"And the trips to the University. Every Wednesday. An hour there, two hours on the court, an hour back. We did that for years."

"We did. With my work and your school, it made for a long day. I enjoyed it and it helped you become a better player."

"I don't think Coach Torne liked me."

"I don't think he liked any one. But, he knew tennis."

"He liked you. He spent as much time talking to you as instructing me."

"He was just explaining what he was doing and letting me know what I could do when he wasn't there."

"He was complicated. Too sophisticated for me. Over my head. I'm not sure I picked up much of what he said."

"You did. Why do you think you got so good?"

"You."

Paul smiled. He contributed to Lauren's success, but knew other coaches had as well, likely more than he had. And he knew the person most entitled to credit was Lauren herself. She worked hard. She was committed and played, played and played. The palms of her right hand were hard with calluses and her knees reworked by orthopedists who repaired damage caused by too many hours of play. In spite of the pain, she worked and worked and worked. She loved it and knew her dad loved it. She worked for both of them. Paul appreciated her effort, her focus, her willing to do what it took, for her, for him, for both of them.

"I don't deserve the credit. You do."

"Thanks, but you were always there, always prodding, always cheering."

Paul was always there; he always cheered. At local tournaments, when she was too young to compete, but competed, he was there and cheered. When she began winning those tournaments, he was there and cheered. Six state tournaments, four-years of collegiate tennis and the USTA, he was there and cheered. When she retired from competitive tennis at 22, he put his hand on a slumped shoulder and with his free hand, massaged a neck that supported a head hung and covered with a towel. She knew it was over and cried. Paul cried as well, but he didn't think she knew, her eyes were closed and shielded by cotton.

"Did you know I cried when your last match ended?"

"Of course. I think you cried more than me."

"How'd you know? You covered your head with a towel."

"I could feel the drops as they hit the towel. I could see the pools of tears on the court. I could feel you shake and hear your sobs."

"Sure."

"I just knew Dad. I knew it was as important to you as it was to me. I knew it was over and knew that a page had been turned. Our Sunday mornings at the courts were over. It wasn't so much that we wouldn't play and plan for competitions again. It wasn't that I wouldn't play high school or college again. It was, that stage in **my** life was over. No, it was, that stage in **our** lives was over. I was no longer your little girl on the tennis court, the blonde with a ponytail, a big racquet and hopes shared with you. I knew we'd never step on the court again, as we had. That's what made me cry and I knew it made you cry too."

"You're right."

Paul was at his office and the courthouse weekdays. He never liked practicing law, because he believed it required him to be a sceptic, a cynic and a jerk. He challenged everything that was presented. *Not true. Not precise enough. Not the right answer.*

The law was adversarial and he was a good lawyer, an adversary's adversary. He didn't like himself when he challenged a colleague, cross-examined an adverse party or ended a conversation with, *We'll see you in Court*. He was conciliatory by nature, but the legal system had changed him, at least from 8:00 until 5:00 weekdays. When he was a young lawyer, he advised clients to compromise, to guard against the all-or-nothing of the courtroom, but when clients determined that caution was a sign of weakness and he saw a misguided superior advocate in the courtroom, with passion, without legal authority, lose and watched the clients who lost, return, more impressed with the passion than hurt by the loss, he morphed. He made a lot of money doing what clients wanted, standing and arguing on their behalf, win or lose.

Tennis with Lauren was an escape from adversity. On the courts, there was him, Lauren, tennis balls, a net and racquets. No arguments, no posturing, no hypocritical final statements, no bruising cross examinations, no sand-papered, vulnerable direct testimony, no judges with incredulous stares. Just tennis. Just father and daughter and tennis. It was escapism of the best sort. His daughter became a good tennis player, but more importantly, a good person. Paul became a proud tennis-father, but more importantly, a good father.

"You're right. I cried. But they were tears of melancholy joy."

"I know Dad. Mine were as well. When I reflect on my life, tennis is prominent. I loved being the little girl with the powerful strokes. I loved playing, I loved winning, but most of all, I loved being with you. I'm glad we did it together."

"I am too."

Slurred by powerful pain medicine, Paul closed his eyes and slept. His waking hours were waking minutes. They were pleasant, but short. He dreamed.

Lauren won the State Championship and when a local reporter asked her what her secret to success was, she said, "My dad." She won the NCAA Division One Singles Championship, and when an ESPN reported asked her to account for her success, she said, "My dad." While standing on a grass court, holding the Wimbledon Trophy, after bowing to the Duchess of Kent and acknowledging the raucous fans, Lauren, with tears in her eyes said, "This is for my Dad, my hero."

Paul woke long enough to discover that Lauren was gone and he was smiling. *Thank God for the drugs. I chose the right option.* He returned to sleep, to England, to the Championships at Wimbledon. As he slept, he smiled.

chapter four

*P*aul slept for an hour. When his eyes opened, he looked around his world and discovered he was alone. He wasn't on the Moon or in Lithuania, Topeka, Point Barrow or Africa, he was in his bedroom, his prison cell, incarcerated by side-rails and disease. It wasn't so bad, given the options. He could have chosen a nursing home or hospital; he chose his bedroom. White, airy, clean and home, nearer those he loved. *Not bad.*

He wasn't sure if he had slept ten minutes or ten hours or even ten days. The drugs that made his life worth living, the elixirs that banned pain from the conversation, interfered with his internal clock. He would fall asleep without warning, in the middle of the day or the middle of a sentence, and sleep for minutes, hours or days. Before he returned home, while he was adjusting to medication, he fell asleep during a conversation with Mary and when he woke, she was still there. He assumed she had waited while he napped, only to later learn his nap was a three-day sleep, during which time, Mary had eaten nine times, had slept in their bed, at their home, three times, showered four times, brushed her teeth six times and read a 460-page novel written by John Irving. His doctor told him the sleep was necessary, his body was fighting cancer, old age and medicine, and that was tiring, but Paul knew his days were numbered and the number was small, and as a result, he had no interest in sleeping away the little time he had left.

Paul rang the small bell on the tray adjacent to his bed, and within thirty seconds, Belle, a hospice nurse, stood at the end of his bed and asked, "Yes sir?"

"How long have I been sleeping?"

Belle looked at her watch, consulted the laptop on the dresser and said, "About an hour."

"Good."

"Good what?"

"Naps are okay, long sleeps in the daytime aren't."

"Why?"

"I don't have much time. I don't want to spend the little time I have remaining, sleeping."

"I understand, but remember, you need sleep. Sleep is restorative. It helps you fight. The better you sleep, the better you can fight. Don't think of sleep as depriving you of time, but as giving you the strength necessary to live longer, to steal time."

"Insightful. A completely different way to look at it. Sleep more, live longer."

Belle tossed a hand-towel caked with dried mucus, into a large, white, canvas bag and returned from the bathroom with a clean one, that she set on the table next to Paul. She smiled. Paul asked, "Why do you do what you do? It seems to me, it would be depressing."

"I love what I do. It can be depressing. I like most of the terminally ill people I work with. When they die, and they almost always do, it's depressing. But, we all die. We all leave this world. Dying is frightening. My job is rewarding, because it gives me an opportunity to be there when I'm needed most. I can help. I'm going to die, you're going to die. If I can help you pass through the rough and scary time, I'm grateful for having had the opportunity. And dying can be peaceful and joyful. When I see that, I am more optimistic about living my life. It sounds crazy, but it's true. That, and the pay is pretty good and there's very little liability." She laughed and when Paul didn't join the laughter, she explained. "You've lived a good and long life. Cancer invaded, your doctors did what they could, but medicine couldn't fix what ails you. My job is simply to keep you comfortable, so that you have an opportunity to say *Goodbye*, with a smile on your face. I feel blessed to be able to do that. We're all terminal, so my job is just to help a fellow traveler."

"Thank you for what you do. And you're right, it is frightening."

"You're not alone. All of my patients are scared. It goes with the territory."

"I went to church as a child, was confirmed and sat in a pew almost every Sunday, until I was diagnosed. I heard all of the things the Pastor said about eternal life, about not deserving it, but receiving it, because I am a Christian child of God. I said the prayers, affirmed my faith proclaiming my right to everlasting, heavenly life, but when you get right down to it, I'm not so sure. I like what I've had here. I'd like it to continue forever. I'm not so sure I'll like what comes hereafter. And that's scary. Damn scary."

"Your faith is being tested. Everyone's is."

"Will I fade to darkness? Will I know I have? Will I find my Mom waiting for me? Will I meet all those people who passed before me? Will they look like they did on their twenty-first birthday or the day they died? Have they been scrubbed clean of imperfections or have their faults followed them to the next stage, and if they are without faults, are they really the people I want to know? My great-grandfather was an abusive drunk. On the other side, is he sober, sensitive and gentle? If he is, is he really my great-grandfather?"

Belle didn't answer with words. She didn't have the answer in words. No one did. Her answer was articulate, empathetic and kind. Her answer was a smile.

"And when you're dead, you're dead. People who've experienced near death, haven't been dead. They didn't go to the place from which they couldn't return. They returned. They weren't dead. So, we have no accounts of what it's like on the other side. I wish we did, but we don't."

"But, those who leave for a while and return, are no longer afraid. Some are drawn to a bright, calming light, others see their lost relatives, but all seem to experience an overwhelming peace. After they've been gone and returned, they're no longer afraid of death. They know something we don't and that something they know has brought them an unwavering confidence that death is beautiful, not horrific."

"But, they returned. Dead is being gone and not returning. It's irreversible. My mother is dead, so is my dad and Abraham Lincoln. They left and didn't return. They're dead. Those who saw a bright light or their departed grandmother and returned, weren't really dead. Does the light dim? Does Grandmother disappear? We don't know, and it's the unknown that's frightening. It's worse not knowing, than knowing the worst. Dreading enlightenment is worse than devastating news."

"Huh?"

"I felt out-of-sorts for months. Just not right. I knew something was wrong, but didn't know what. I avoided doctors. I refused to look in mirrors, fearing I'd see something that would reveal the cause of my angst. I didn't touch myself in certain places, afraid if I did, I'd discover a lump. I was obsessed with my symptoms and scared damn near to death, that they would lead me to a deadly diagnosis. Cancer? Aneurisms? Deadly auto-immune diseases? Incurable deadly virus? I was in a constant state of fret. When the pain became unbearable, when I couldn't breathe, when it was unavoidable, I went to the doctor. Within days, I was diagnosed with Stage IV lung cancer. Incurable? Yup. Deadly? Yup. But the strange thing is, knowing was much better than not knowing. Even though I learned the symptoms that scared me revealed a deadly disease, I was relieved to know. Not knowing is the worst."

"Realizing your worst fears was better than the fear of the unknown?"

"Yup. Anticipating the worst is the worst. A diagnosis is concrete, real. When you know what it is, you can take the next step. Treatment, surrender. Doesn't matter which, it's a place to be, a direction in which to move. No floundering, no ignorance based fears. Knowing is better, even if the knowledge received isn't what you were looking for."

"How long have you believed that?"

"A long time. When I was eight, my best friend's dad walked into his living room in a robe. He stooped to pick up the newspaper and his robe opened, revealing a gnarly twelve-inch scar that looked like a flattened bull snake. When he saw I was scared, he tried to calm my fears by saying, *Paul, it's a scar from surgery I had when I was young. I swallowed a bug and surgery was necessary to make me healthy again.* Years later, I determined he had swallowed a tuberculosis germ and he called it a bug so I'd better understand, but then, I had no idea. Later that day, the day he told me he had swallowed a bug, his son and I were playing basketball in his backyard and while I was still obsessing about the scar, I jumped high for a rebound, took a deep breath and sucked a fly down my throat. I tried unsuccessfully to cough it up and spit it out, but it was all inevitable to me. I lifted my shirt and pictured a flattened bull snake wrapped around my little, hairless, thin, torso and walked home. I told no one; I wasn't interested in treatment, treatment meant diagnosis, surgery and a bull-snake wrapped around my belly. So, I suffered in silence.

"A week later, my Mom went shopping and I tagged along. We stopped at an arcade and I spotted a machine that promised to tell me my future for a penny. It was called *"Your Destiny, Your Horoscope."* I had no idea what *destiny* or *horoscope* meant, but I was burdened and wanted to relieve myself with a map of my future, so I asked my Mom for a penny and dropped it in the slot. Before the machine could provide me with the relief I sought, it required that I dial in my birthdate, which, with help from my Mom, I was able to do. *July 21.* After the machine received the requested information, lights flashed and the mechanical sooth-sayer grumbled in its metal guts and ultimately, with a great deal of fanfare, spit a small piece of paper, on which was printed my future. With trembling hands, in need of peace, I reached for my horoscope and in large block letters, on the top and in the middle, read, **CANCER**.

"There were more words on the small white strip of paper, but I had read enough. I was eight. I had no idea that people born in mid-July were assigned the astrological sign *Cancer*. I thought it was confirmation of my suspicions. I went for a rebound, swallowed a bug, dropped a penny in the slot and black-magically, *Cancer*.

"When I was younger, I'd get an upset stomach and think I had stomach cancer. I'd get heart-burn and panic, thinking I was having a heart attack. A bruise? Internal bleeding. A cough? Lung cancer. Difficulty urinating? Bladder cancer. A rash? Skin cancer. I'd wait for the symptoms to disappear on their own, and often they did. When they didn't go away, and got worse, I'd go to the doctor, he'd give me an anti-biotic or topical, I'd swallow and apply and the symptoms would disappear. Every time, I'd call myself an idiot for waiting and fretting and vow to keep it in perspective in the future and see a doctor as soon as I had questions. So, I've known for a long time."

"You poor boy."

"It was a long time ago. I should've learned my lesson."

"And yet, when the symptoms suggested sickness months ago, you fretted and worried in ignorance?"

"Yup. Can't say why, except to blame it on a scar and a horoscope machine. I learned the lesson, but didn't implement it. I don't know why. I worried about a bug morphing into a physical scar snaking across my distended belly. I should have been worried about emotional scars. The bug I swallowed wasn't responsible for my cancer, it was however, responsible for how I reacted to cancer's symptoms. It created emotional scars. I guess I was just waiting for the symptoms to go away on their own. Worry, hoping, worrying."

Belle smiled and said a silent prayer for her patient. Her lips moved, but sound didn't escape her mouth.

Paul wasn't certain how to react to the silent prayer. He assumed it was about and for him. It engendered two, opposite responses. He was modestly offended that Belle believed she had powers Paul didn't possess, that she could do what he couldn't. The overly, overtly religious. Sticking their noses where they don't belong. He was sick, not helpless, not incapable of lobbying for his own peace, his pleasant hereafter. He was modestly offended, but at the same time, appreciative that Belle would do what she could to help him. The benevolent believers, trying to help when and where they can. She was intervening on his behalf, using her political capital with the man-in-charge, the gatekeeper,

God. He rejected offended, recognizing it was driven by a fragile ego, ill-health and vanity, and settled on appreciation. "Thank you for your prayers."

Belle's lips continued to move while her eyes were closed. She had heard Paul, knew he had thanked her, but completed her conversation with one more important than Paul, before she responded. When her lips stopped moving, she looked to the ceiling, crossed herself, looked at Paul and answered a question not asked. "You are deserving of God's grace and I'm glad I can help."

"Do you have doubts?"

"Sometimes. Everyone does. I'm not always certain, and can't tell you that I would be if I were in that bed, in your condition. I like to think I would be, but I've been around long enough to see the most faithful, lose faith." She looked to the ceiling and beyond, before she continued. Although she didn't say, Paul knew she was asking that her faith remain strong, that she not drift as others had. "So, I'll keep doing the best I can, knowing I can't do it alone."

Paul admired Belle's faith. He'd never had faith. *Too logical. Too smart. Too vain.* When he was 25, he had an argument with a friend. It was civil. No one swore, no one shouted. Paul's friend, an agnostic, refused to investigate religion, believing it was simply a tool used by the powerful to keep the masses in line. *No proof, no faith*, he said. Paul argued that there was no upside to being a non-believer, and that even in the absence of proof, he'd maintain at least a semblance of faith, because there was always an upside to being a believer. *If there is no God, there is no negative consequence for believing, but if there is one, and faith in that God is rejected, there could be some pretty scary consequences. No sense in not believing. There's no benefit.*

So, Paul went to church, said his prayers, baptized his children and donated money to the Church. When he mumbled the *Apostle's Creed* with the congregation, saying he believed in the life everlasting, he wasn't sure, but calculated there was no harm in saying so. When his young children asked him about dying, he told them Jesus would save their souls and they would live in Heaven forever, because maybe it was true and there was no downside to his kids believing in Jesus and accepting that he was the path to everlasting life, but he wasn't sure what he said was true. He tried to find faith, an internal and abiding belief in something he couldn't see, feel or prove, but was unable to find it. "I envy you. I wish I had your faith."

"When you need it, it will be there."

"I hope so." But he wasn't sure.

"Trust me." Belle smiled, believing she had said something important, done something even more important, had witnessed for Christianity. Her smile was not ego-driven. She didn't feel self-important, didn't swell with selfish pride, believing her place or faith made her better than Paul; she smiled because she believed she had helped a wandering man find refuge and a shot at peace.

Belle stood, adjusted Paul's I.V., refreshed his water glass with cold water and ice, adjusted his pillow and asked, "When you get there, will you tell me? Send me a sign? I think I'm right, feel it in my soul, but it would be nice to know from someone who's there."

"I asked my Mom to do the same."

"And?"

"Still waiting. Nothing. Silence. Her picture fell from the wall while we were eating Christmas dinner two weeks after she died and the car I inherited from her burst into flames on the first anniversary of her death, but I don't think either was a message from the grave."

"Likely not. I want my message to be more articulate, absolutely clear, in English. Call me on the phone, send a postcard from Heaven, seize control of my television and send programing from the other side. Be clear."

"I'll try. What's your address and phone number?"

Paul laughed, as did Belle, but when Paul's laugh triggered a deep, phlegm-filled cough, their smiles vanished. Belle moved Paul's back from the bed, attempting to open his air passage-ways and quiet the cough and when she did, the coughing jag ended. She smiled and said, "I'll write them down so you can study them and not forget them when the time is right. It may be a while."

While they both smiled, Paul closed his eyes and drifted to sleep.

When Paul woke, an hour or a day later, he opened his eyes and through the fog of pain-medication and deep sleep, peered through the window of his bedroom into a world of darting squirrels, loud, black crows, bird-feeders, green grass, trimmed bushes and lawnmowers. A strong wind blew from the west and the oak trees, full of leaves, leaned to the east, revealing what they block from view on a still day. Two miles from his home, across the Rum River and Main Street in Anoka, Paul saw a church steeple, and resting on its peak, oblivious to the wind, standing tall and resolute, a barren cross. It was Paul's Church and the Cross that had welcomed him on Sundays for more than 60-years. It welcomed him again. He smiled, closed his eyes, but did not sleep. He smiled, his lips moved, but he did not speak. He smiled, he prayed and then he slept.

chapter five

When the wind stopped, the trees stood tall and Paul, awake after another nap, craned his skinny neck, but was no longer able to see his Church. *Tomorrow. If there is tomorrow. And if not, if today is all I have here, I can't see it, but I know it's still here.*

Paul thought he heard a familiar voice, a man's voice. He heard Mary laugh and the familiar voice spoke again, and Mary laughed again. He was the one who was dying, the one the familiar voice came to see, yet Mary was having all the fun. *Not fair, not right.* Paul rang his bell.

Cliff Snell, the former agnostic with whom Paul had a civil disagreement about the value of having faith 60-years earlier, the man Paul told there was no harm in believing if what you believed was a fiction, but that hell could be the consequence if you didn't believe and what you denied was real, walked into the bedroom, wearing shorts, tennis shoes, a Tee-shirt inscribed with, *Don't Mess With the Old Man, He Might Just Die* and a smile. As Cliff gently reached for Paul's shrinking paw,

Paul snickered and asked, "Why are *you* wearing a shirt made for me?"

Cliff buried his chin in his chest, lifted cotton from flesh and read his shirt. He blushed. "Sorry. I shoulda dressed more carefully."

"That's okay. I wore an *I'm With Stupid* tee-shirt, with Mary, on our thirtieth anniversary. So, I know inappropriate tee-shirts."

"How'd that happen?"

"Mary and I went grocery shopping, to buy food for an anniversary dinner at home, and the cashier asked if my better-half approved of my shirt. I looked at what I wore, like you, blushed, and said *Ooops*. I know inappropriate tee-shirts."

Lauren had bought the *I'm With Stupid* tee-shirt for Paul on his sixtieth birthday. A gag-gift. When Paul opened the gift, removed the shirt and read the words printed on its front, he asked, *Why'd you buy your mom a tee-shirt on my birthday?* He wore it on summer Saturdays and Sundays, because it was light weight, gray, a color that looked good on Paul when his face was flush with sun, had a good collar that fit snuggly over his old man neck and he rarely read what was written between his nipples. On their thirtieth anniversary, until the cashier interrupted the celebrating couple's ignorance, Mary hadn't noticed what was written on Paul's chest. She smiled at the moderately offended cashier and said nothing to Paul. When they returned home from the store, understanding he would soon be sitting across the kitchen table, sharing an anniversary meal *with stupid*, Paul changed shirts.

"How do you feel my friend?"

Always sensitive, always concerned, always sincere. Cliff was Paul's best friend, had been for 70-years. They walked to kindergarten together, drove to high school together, skipped school to smoke cigarettes in a 1946 Chevrolet together, joined the Army together and after discharge, lived together in a musty apartment on the second floor of a building that housed a furniture store, in Anoka. When Paul returned to the United States after 12-months in Viet Nam, Cliff who served his hitch in the Army on a base on the East Coast, flew to Ft. Lewis, Washington to meet Paul. Together, not often alone.

"I'm okay. Better than I was at Ft. Lewis. I'm dying now. Then, I think I was dead."

Cliff smiled, then frowned as he returned to 1965 and remembered decades-old vacant stares, hollow cheeks, silence and dread. "You were lost."

"I'm glad you were there to find me. But you're right. I was lost."

The return flight, the plane trip that brought young soldiers home from Vietnam, a commercial Pan Am flight, was known as the *Freedom Flight*. It was supposed to be liberating, fun, relaxing, an escape hatch for the weary, a new beginning for those who didn't have the money, position or luck to avoid the draft and those who were fortunate enough to escape death in a field of rice. It was a trip from terror to home, a trip from Vietnam to Ft. Lewis, Washington. Although the passengers had dreamed of the *Freedom Flight*, anticipated its arrival and their departure, it was none of what it was supposed to be. It wasn't liberating, fun or relaxed.

As the plane sat on the tarmac in Da Nang, South Vietnam, the passengers were pensive, quiet, breathing little, if at all, waiting to be in the air, over the ocean, out of range. When the plane reached safety, the pilot announced that it had left Vietnam, Paul expected to hear hoopla, a celebration, but no one said anything. They sat in their seats, waiting for it to be over. As the plane landed in the Philippines, they waited. When the place landed and left Hawaii, they waited and when the plane touched down in the continental United States, at Ft. Lewis, they were still waiting. Paul wondered if some were still waiting.

"Yeah, it was strange. They didn't do it right. The Army, 200 years of tradition, unspoiled by progress. Not very smart, especially in 65. We were in the jungle one day, and after a couple of long flights, we were on the streets of home the next day. No transition, no debriefing, no decompression, just *Get the fuck out.*" Paul grinned at his word choice. Around the children and Mary and in the office, he rarely cussed and never said *fuck*. But, after a short metaphysical trip to 1965, wearing an imaginary helmet, camouflage and wet boots filled with squishy socks and blistered toes, it was ..*Get the fuck out.*

"It was ironic. Different from our arrival. When we flew to Vietnam, we were on our way to war, but there was an excitement, an optimism, on the plane. I flew with guys I trained with and we happily yakked as we crossed the Pacific on our way to combat. We were tough; we were ready. On the way to war, we had fun and during our escape from war, on the *Freedom Flight* home, we were so scarred by war, we couldn't enjoy our deliverance."

"I wish I could have been there with you."

Cliff felt guilt. Had for more than 50 years. He was haunted by the sacrifice of others. Late at night, when the television screen was black and the radio silent, while his wife and children slept, when he paged through his high school yearbook and made note of those who went and those who lost, he cried. *I'm responsible.*

Others died. Others survived, but were changed by war. They lost limbs, innocence, hope. Others were scarred by Agent Orange, shrapnel and fear, while Cliff shuffled papers at Ft. Lee, Virginia. They died and struggled to survive, escaped battle haunted by what they did and did not do, while Cliff sat on comfortable leather chairs, in an air-conditioned office and shuffled papers. He could have done more. He shouldn't have slept between crisp white sheets on a comfortable mattress while they slept in the jungle, trying to avoid snipers, booby-traps and rain. It wasn't fair that they gave so much, while Cliff gave so little. Not fair at all. He cried. *I'm responsible.*

After Randy was born, Cliff and Paul met to celebrate his birth at the Anoka VFW. Cliff parked on First Avenue, in front of the VFW and under a cloudless sky, waited in his car for Paul. When Paul arrived wearing a broad smile, holding cigars wrapped in cellophane, emblazoned with, *It's a Boy,* they walked into the dark windowless club. The VFW was hot and humid and garnished with the smell of sweet liquor and stale vomit, when Paul and Cliff celebrated Randy's arrival. Former soldiers, men who sat at the bar and stared into glasses mixed with pain, regret and beer, broken veterans who served overseas and said nothing, except, *Another*, looked away from their glasses, nodded at the newcomers and returned to brood in beer.

Cliff sat at a Formica table, cleaned its dirty top with a napkin, and said, "You know why I waited? You know why I didn't come in and wait for you in here? I'm not a member. I can't join the VFW. I didn't serve overseas."

After four pitchers of beer and three shots of whiskey, Cliff said, "You know why I can't join the VFW? I didn't serve overseas."

"I know. You said that before."

Cliff surveyed the room adorned with pictures of Iwo Jima, the Forrestal, American flags, Purple Hearts, empty uniforms and shrouded in the desolation of its members and cried. Paul watched, but said nothing. It wasn't the first time, and times before Paul had intervened and actively tried to dry Cliff's tears, and failed. He knew the best answer was time and silence, an opportunity for Cliff to sort it out, to salve the wound germinated in a state-side incubator and festered in guilt dressed by the pain of others, the pain of men who served overseas and were eligible to join the VFW. Cliff cried.

Kismet. Cliff had done nothing to shield himself from battle. He volunteered to serve in the Army and asked to go to paratrooper's school, knowing if his request was granted, he'd have been in Vietnam within six-months of graduation. The Army recognized Cliff's intelligence, concluded that making him a paratrooper would fail to take advantage of his smarts, and trained him as an Administrative Support Specialist. While Paul walked through swamps, carrying an M-16 and searching for booby-traps, while he dried his boots and socks over fires that burned while temperatures hovered near 100 degrees, while Paul met Vietnamese women in small dirty bars in Saigon, Cliff kept track of earnings statements and leave balances just outside of Richmond, Virginia.

When Cliff stopped crying, after he disappeared into the bathroom and returned to the barroom with a sheepish smile, embarrassed by the revelation, Paul consoled his lifelong friend. "Be glad that you weren't there. It wasn't pleasant. Look at these guys."

"But I should have shared the suffering of my generation, and I didn't. It's not right that they suffered while I shuffled paper."

"Wasn't your choice my friend. As I recall, you volunteered for Nam and I didn't. I was reluctant; you were willing."

"Maybe you should have volunteered and I shouldn't have. Maybe I'd have gone and you'd have stayed home."

"It doesn't matter now. We did what we were asked to do. And we lost anyway."

"Maybe had I been there, we'd have won." He chuckled, bringing splotches of red to his balding dome. He lifted a glass, smiled and said, "To Randy and to all these brave men, including you."

Cliff removed his tee-short by pulling it over his head, reversed it and put it back on, covering his torso with an inside-out tee that couldn't be read. He gripped the side-rails of Paul's bed and said, "Better?"

Paul answered with a smile and Cliff asked, "Do you have regrets?"

"About Vietnam?"

"No, about life."

Paul had asked himself that same question after the Doctor told him he would soon be dead. He asked, because he wanted to leave with a clear conscience and knew he had little time to make things right. The answer he gave himself was different than the one he'd give Cliff. The answer he gave himself would remain his secret. He had regrets, but he wouldn't share those regrets with anyone, not Cliff, especially, not Mary.

Before the Doctor disappeared, soon after telling Paul he carried cancer in his lungs, while Paul laid on a hospital bed with tears falling from his face to a starched, white pillow case, as he accepted his mortality and asked himself about regrets, the answer appeared. He didn't need to prepare a list and prioritize indiscretions. He didn't need to wake a sleepy, forgotten memory. He didn't need to choose. It was clear. He didn't need to wait long for the answer. It was clear.

In Kentucky, in 1973, two years after Mary gave birth to Lauren, while on a business trip, Paul met Lisa Carnes. Lisa was 56 years old, Paul, 33. Lisa was the owner of a manufacturing company she had inherited from her father. Lisa's company manufactured sprockets that were used on Indian motorcycles. On a rural road in northern Minnesota, in June, 1969, a sprocket manufactured by Lisa's company malfunctioned, and Dave Drayer, driving an Indian, fell to the pavement and died when he slid into a telephone pole planted in dirt on the side of the road. The law firm for whom Paul worked sued Lisa's Company, *Specialty Sprockets,* and Paul was sent to Lexington, Kentucky, to depose Lisa.

The deposition was uneventful. Lisa had no answers to the questions Paul asked. Almost one-hundred times, she said, "I'm sorry, I don't know. My involvement with the Company is limited to its finances and the operation of the Board of Directors. I know nothing particular about the manufacturing of sprockets."

She was pleasant. Unlike other opposing parties Paul had deposed, she didn't snarl or bite. She smiled, read her answer from a card given to her by her lawyer, and patiently waited for the next question. When the deposition was over and the court reporter had gathered her equipment and left Paul, Lisa and Lisa's lawyer in the conference room alone, Lisa apologized for her inability to shed light on the accident or the malfunction. She seemed sincere, but Paul, a tarnished, cynical, skeptical lawyer, wasn't so sure. He'd been convinced by the insincere before and recognized his inability to always divine the truth.

"Would you like to get lunch?" Lisa directed her question to Paul and her lawyer, who declined the offer, explaining he had work to do and a hearing early that afternoon.

Paul said, "Why not?"

They purchased a light lunch at a street kiosk and ate on a bench overlooking a small park. Fifteen minutes after tossing paper plates, napkins and plastic cups in a metal garbage can chained to the side of an office building, Paul and Lisa walked passed a doorman, who tipped his cap and said, "Miss Powell," and took the elevator to the 18th floor. Before the door to Lisa's condominium was completely closed, as the crack created by the door and its frame narrowed, Lisa and Paul kissed. The kiss wasn't polite; it wasn't tentative, waiting for permission to be passionate, it was committed, hot and premonitory.

As the first kiss predicted, Paul and Lisa consummated their affair. She was 56 years old, but resilient like a 22 year old. *Once. Twice. Three times.*

Lisa brought Paul to the airport. When Paul fell asleep that night, in a bed he shared with Mary, across the hall from his daughter, he was erect and consumed by guilt, both spawned by Lisa. He loved Mary, and truth be told, loved Lauren more, but the excitement created by a 56 year old, too old for children and too young for pasture, demanded his attention and compromised his loyalties. He tried to forget, but couldn't.

Paul telephoned Lisa the day after he met her. She was as smitten with the young man as he was with the older woman. Their relationship endured. Whenever Paul was called from home to the road, whether it was Dubuque, Iowa, Denver, Colorado, Hershey, Pennsylvania or Detroit, Michigan, Lisa traveled to where Paul was and they shared each other. Eight times, Lisa visited the Twin Cities, but saw only the airport, the inside of her hotel room and Paul.

The odd couple knew their relationship would travel no further than it had been. It was, like Paul now, confined to a room. There were extenuating circumstances, restrictions to growth that couldn't be avoided. Paul was married to a woman he loved, the mother of his daughter and pregnant with his second child. He was as faithful as an unfaithful man could be. He wasn't looking, he tried to forget. It was unavoidable, demanded by the stars, preordained by the secular gods. It was what it was, and was to remain as it was. Lisa and Paul often talked about it. Usually they laughed.

Sitting up bed, wearing sheets as a turtleneck sweater to hide wrinkles and sagging breasts, smiling, as she seemingly always did, Lisa accepted their plight. "I get it. We'll never have it all. But I like what we have and am unwilling to give it up. If you tell me *No more*, I'll accept that, but if you don't, I'll keep coming back, so long as I can."

Paul, then 36, three years into their relationship, returned her smile and said something he had only said to one person before. "I love you, Lisa."

Once, twice, three times.

In a twisted sense of loyalty, when Mary gave birth to Randy, Paul's son, Paul wanted to share the news with Lisa. He held his newborn baby, kissed his son's mother's forehead and hastily left the hospital, found a public phone and dialed his other lover. Paul found it strange that Lisa didn't answer, she always did, but given the celebration ignited by the birth of his son, it was of minor consequence to Paul.

After beer, tears and conversation with Cliff at the VFW, Paul called Lisa later that evening, and at breakfast time, lunch time and supper time, for the next three days. She didn't answer. *Not three times, not twice, not once.*

Paul told his office he had a family emergency and his wife, an office emergency, and leaving his two children, one not five days old, and his tired new-mother wife, flew to Kentucky. Lisa was dead. She died of an aneurism on the day Randy was born and was buried on the day Paul arrived in Kentucky.

Paul was broken by grief and unable to mend with the help of friends. He suffered in silence, alone. Only one person knew of his divided heart, and she was dead. He was alone. He cried in the shower, so his tears would remain hidden; he shouted insults at God for taking her from him, in the car, with windows closed and the radio playing loudly, so his words would not be heard. He stayed in bed long after the clock told him to rise and when his feet found the floor, his shoulders slouched and his slippers shuffled across the floor. He lost interest and his energy was consumed by grief and unavailable for walking, talking, eating. He lost ten pounds from an already slender frame and increased his intake of nicotine from 45 to 65 cigarettes daily.

He neglected his newborn son, asking Mary to rise when he cried in the night and avoiding dirty diapers and bottles. He had been attentive to Lauren, not so much for Randy. He was a good baby, rarely cried, smiled often and looked a lot like Paul did as a baby. Paul should have been happy, attentive, proud, but he wasn't; he was alone with his grief.

His dour attitude, his inattentiveness, was obvious. Lauren asked, *Are you all right Daddy,* and Mary asked, *What's wrong.*

He dismissed their questions, their concern, with, *I'm fine. Just work, that's all.* But it was more. He was haunted by loss and unable to focus, frame a plan for happiness or force a prolonged smile for nearly a year.

A year after Lisa's death, Paul received a bonus check, his share of money received in a settlement acquired for Dave Drayer's widow, from *Specialty Sprockets*. The check was larger than Paul expected and he was surprised, believing it would not be paid until after a trial scheduled to begin eight months later. When he asked, he was told, "The old woman who owned the Company died. No husband, no kids. Lots of cousins. The estate wasn't interested in a lawsuit. It wanted it over, so it could distribute money to the heirs, 21 of them I understand. So, we settled. It was a pretty good deal for Mrs. Drayer."

Old woman? She wasn't old and Paul was offended by the accusation that belittled a woman he loved and the pain he carried. He cashed the check, used the proceeds to purchase furniture, equipment and an office lease and opened his own firm, a firm that remained open in downtown Anoka, a firm in a building with a large corner office, which was filled with paper, furniture, pictures and memories, but now unoccupied, in respect for the dying.

Paul loved Lisa, but regretted that he gave his heart to another while married to a woman he loved. He had never told anyone about Lisa, but missed her terribly for the year after she died. At night, when he laid in bed and asked for direction and forgiveness, he spoke to God and Lisa, not Mary. He felt terrible about violating his vows to Mary, but felt worse about falling in love with a woman who loved him and was unable to love him in the way she wanted, openly. Paul carried guilt for years. He was upset with himself for depriving Mary of his undivided love, but was consumed by guilt for denying Lisa an open, committed, loving, relationship, a relationship that could have completed her life. Before falling asleep, every night for the year following Lisa's death, Paul ended his prayer with, *I'm so sorry Lisa.*

Paul's grief was slowly consumed by time. He didn't remember when it ended; it wasn't an exclamation point following a defined period of time. When his third child, Alyson, was born, Paul attended to her dirty diapers, bottles and rose at night to quiet her. As he silently rocked her in the dark, he thought of Lisa, whispered, *You should have known Lisa, she was amazing*, and with his admission to a child who cooed but did not comprehend, recognized that grief no longer plagued him. He missed Lisa, but it had found perspective.

During the 39 years between Lisa's death and Paul's diagnosis, he was often visited by guilt and shame. When a politician was accused of infidelity and Mary called him *scum*, Paul felt guilty. When Randy asked if he was a difficult, colicky child, if he needed attention in the middle of the night, Paul felt guilty for his neglect, and in the interest of amends, took him to a ball game or gave him an extra-long hug. When divorce clients confessed their affairs, and explained discovery had ended their marriage, Paul felt guilty for his indiscretion, but lucky that discovery had been avoided and his marriage was strong and intact.

It was complicated. He felt blessed to have loved Lisa, but was ashamed of what he had done. It was his one regret.

Paul looked at Cliff, determined he was waiting for an answer and answered as best he could, without revealing the truth. "We all have regrets. I'm no different. Nothing I can do now. I've made peace."

Paul wondered if Lisa would be on the other side, and if so, would she recognize him? He'd grown old and small. His hair was nearly gone, his muscles atrophied and his erection, something they both loved, a memory. If she was there, if they recognized each other, on the other side, would they need to hide their passions, and if not, what would happen to those passions when Mary joined them, on the other side, in the hereafter?

"Want me to leave so you can get some sleep."

"No. I'm not tired. Just drifting to another time."

"1957?" It was when Paul and Cliff graduated high school.

"No, but I'm happy to go there. It was a good year."

"It was. A 1946 Chevrolet and a bottle of Tequila."

Cliff was a good friend, with an agenda. He knew what he was supposed to be doing, at the bed of a dying man. He understood the power of memory, the palliative potential of reflection.

"I remember."

"As I recall, you had a hard time with the clutch sober and when you drank alcohol, you were completely incapable."

Paul remembered. He was right, but Paul was unwilling to confess to a weakness behind the wheel. What self-respecting 17 year old would? "I was born with a talent for driving and a little tequila never compromised my God-given talents."

"Well then, how do you explain a charred transmission and warped clutch plate in a 1946 Chevy with an empty tequila bottle in the backseat?"

Paul had no credible explanation. The recently graduated 17-year olds celebrated graduation by stealing a bottle of tequila from Paul's dad, who drank enough to not miss a bottle or two, and drove a dirt road to Emily Skinner's house. Emily and June Sparks joined the boys and they drove country roads, minimum maintenance roads, while drinking stolen tequila. Paul let the clutch out too slowly when sober, and when drunk, rode it mercilessly. From a stop, the inebriate lifted his left foot, allowing the clutch pedal to rise, but as the car moved forward, Paul kept the pedal partially depressed, sending a contradictory message to the Chevy, *move, don't move.*

On that day in June, 1957, the roads were full of ruts, which required frequent changes of pace, which meant Paul was constantly moving the clutch pedal up and down. Cliff warned him to lift his foot completely off the clutch or risk burning it, but either the words were too slurred to be understood or Paul was simply too drunk to understand, so the message went unheeded. Twenty-minutes after Emily jumped in the front seat and June in the back, four miles from tar, the driver and passengers smelled something burning and when Paul tried to shift gears, heard clunking, grinding and rubber locking stationary on gravel. The

Chevy stopped and despite Paul's best efforts, it wouldn't move. They were 17, drunk, stranded and far from home. At the time, Paul accepted responsibility, "Sorry guys. My fault."

Fifty-eight years later, dying, smiling, manipulating history, Paul rejected responsibility. "I wasn't drunk and never rode the clutch. I think that transmission was on its way to the junk heap before we popped the cork on that bottle of tequila."

"Mr. Skinner didn't think so. When he tied the car to his tractor with a chain used to pull stumps, he took a whiff of the air near that broken Chevy and said, *Somebody's been riding a clutch.*"

"He was a farmer, not a mechanic."

They talked about Cliff's wife, who died two years earlier of a heart attack. She hadn't sent a sign from the other side, but Cliff thought she'd be happy to see Paul, absent a miracle. They talked about the law, how Paul had never enjoyed practicing it and how Cliff had never been satisfied with the results it provided when someone accused his business of not keeping its end of the bargain. They remembered classmates who died and lamented failing memories, aching joints, growing mid-drifts and disappearing energy and passion. When Cliff stood to leave, he put his hands over Paul's diminished paws and asked, "Is there anything I can do?"

There was. And Paul told him.

chapter
six

After giving Cliff instructions, Paul slept. As he slept, he dreamed of his friend, someone he'd seen almost daily for nearly 70 years. In his dream, they were on a ballfield, a dance floor, an airplane, in a theater, a '46 Chevy and trouble. Cliff was always joking, always grinning, always fixing what had gone wrong, with a kind word and an apology. When Paul's eyes opened, visions from his dream remained and he thought he saw Cliff at the end of his bed. It wasn't Cliff, it was Mary. She smiled.

"Has Cliff left?"

"Yup. All gone. I'm sure he'll be back."

"I had a Cliff dream. It made me remember. I want to tell him."

"Tell me."

"You wouldn't understand. You weren't there."

"Try me. Bring me there."

Paul was a storyteller. His kids pulled up a chair when he started to spin a yarn, knowing it would be a while and if they stood for the tale, their legs would weaken, then buckle. He remembered the details and recounted them colorfully in an attempt to make his stories come alive. His grandchildren, six fresh faces to whom Paul had said *Goodbye* when he was in the hospital, a dozen lovely children Paul had excluded from his bedroom, his hospice, wanting them to remember him as he had been, not as a 95 pound frail and pasty sick man, encouraged him to regale them with stories of the days when Papa and Nama were young, when televisions showed black and white pictures and waste wasn't flushed, but rather buried with black dirt and a shovel. *Please Papa, tell us a story. Please.*

Mary looked at her husband and wanted him to tell while he could. She didn't ask her Mother, and then, she was dead. She hadn't asked her Father, and then he was dead. Paul was alive; she'd not fail to ask him as she had her Mother and Father. "Please Papa, tell me that story."

Never able to ignore the pleas of his grandchildren, Paul grinned at his resourceful wife who had channeled the grandkids, convincing Paul to do what he had declined to do when the request was made simply by Mary. She was clever, wise beyond her years or perhaps, wise to her years and so, Paul told Mary the story he had wanted to tell Cliff.

"In 1965, Cliff and I spent a weekend in Tacoma. He met me when the plane delivered me from Vietnam. I wasn't good company. I was only 30 hours from battle and hadn't learned how to relax. Cliff anticipated that I'd be out of sorts, and guessed I'd used drugs in Vietnam, and decided a little marijuana might be what I needed and expected upon my arrival in the States.

"I'd used a little marijuana while in Vietnam, but it wasn't very potent. Most of the time, I needed to add alcohol to feel anything. I'm guessing the drugs we found in Vietnam were cut with tobacco, weakened, because our dealers, other soldiers, knew we couldn't stay alive if we were completely out of our minds on drugs. So, in Vietnam, we smoked a little, drifted a little, smoked some more, buzzed a little and slept. No big deal.

"The stuff that Cliff had, he bought from a friend who claimed it had been delivered to him by a guy who was discharged from the Army in Vietnam, but stayed in Asia after his discharge, to see that part of the continent not ravaged by war. According to Cliff, the marijuana he brought to Tacoma was from Thailand and was the *good stuff.*

"We rented a car and drove towards Puget Sound. As we drove, we smoked the marijuana Cliff had carried with him from Virginia. Because the marijuana worked and worked fast, we didn't make it to the water, but instead stopped in downtown Tacoma. We walked to a park and sat on a bench while the grass we smoked distorted our perceptions. It was weird, almost frightening. As I inhaled, I wanted to expel the potentially poisonous gases and when my eyes closed, my lids banged together more loudly than a car door closed by an angry man. It was weird, almost frightening. It was dark and the only light came from passing cars and streetlights. Cliff suggested we walk and I agreed, hoping the dope's power would be diminished in the event we stood and burned energy as we walked. It wasn't.

"I remember walking in the direction of a street light and no matter how many steps I took, I never got any closer to that light. I walked to the lamp for what seemed like a half-an-hour, and yet remained as far from the lamp as I had been when I separated my ass from the park bench. We were too stoned to drive and it was getting a bit cool, so we decided to go to a movie house down the block. It was showing *Doctor Zhivago*.

"It seemed as though it took us days to walk down the block to the theater, but eventually, without stopping for food, water or sleep, we paid either five-dollars or five-hundred dollars for our tickets and entered the theater. I asked the man in the ticket booth how long the movie was and was told it almost three-and-a-half hours. I was okay with that, because I was so wasted, I knew I needed a large block of time to sober up and be able to drive.

"When the Coming Attractions were over, I turned to the back of the theater to determine the time and estimate the time the movie would end. A clock with numbers and arms illuminated in red, said it was 8:15, and after miscalculating the additional three-and-a-half hours, three times, I settled on an end time of 11:45. And the movie began.

"It was epic. Sand, camels, Arabs, wind, tents and dialogue I had a hard time following. And so long. I was expecting the credits, the end, so many times, I lost count. So, long. Interminably long. Insufferably long. It wouldn't end. I began to despise the camels, Omar Sharif and even Julie Christie. Get to the point. Be done. Too long. Quit wasting my time. Please. As I concluded that I had never experienced so long a three-and-a-half-hour block of time, I turned to look at the clock in the rear of the theater. 11:10? 11:15? Did I miscalculate time while under the influence of drugs and was it midnight? **It was 8:20**. The interminably long movie had started just five minutes earlier. Not three hours, not even two-and-a-half-hours, five minutes. Five flipping minutes."

Mary looked at Paul and waited. She expected there was more, a punchline she would understand, a punchline she could appreciate. She waited and when no more was said, she asked, "And?"

"And? Nothing. That's it."

"Oh." She looked at the iPad on her lap, out the window across the room, moistened her lips with *ChapStick*, adjusted the collar of her shirt and hem of her pants, cleared her throat two times, wiped imaginary sleep from her eyes and, without nothing more to say, repeated herself. "Oh."

"See, I told you, you had to be there. I should have waited for Cliff. He'd understand. He'd appreciate it."

"Did you stay to the end of the movie?"

Frustration grew in Paul's ransacked body. She didn't get it. It was clear. Any man would've understood. Women and men. Cats and dogs. Republicans and Democrats. Unbelievable. "I don't remember if we stayed. It was 45 years ago."

"But, you remember the clock so vividly."

Exasperated. "The clock is an integral part of the story. I need to remember the clock. I don't need to know what we did after

69

believing five minutes was four hours. It's irrelevant. The clock isn't irrelevant, it's important."

"Were you able to drive the car after the movie was over?"

Paul surrendered. His story had missed its mark. It was a failure. "I'm not sure. Let's talk about something else."

"I didn't know you used drugs. Did you often use drugs?" Paul closed his eyes when Mary asked the question. He half-heartedly expected her to end the question with *Archie. I didn't know you used drugs, Archie.*

"That was it, Edith. The one and only time. It was only once."

"Edith?"

"Forget it."

Paul cleared his throat and awakened the pain sensors in his lungs. As Mary began to ask a question, Paul raised his left index finger, asking for a small window of silence, and when it was given, he waited for the pain to pass. It did and he said, "Sorry. What did you want to say?"

"Randy will be here tomorrow."

"Why? Doesn't he work?" Randy was a schoolteacher in Kentucky. He graduated from law school, *Order of the coif*, practiced with a securities law firm in St. Paul, and abandoned the practice of law, to teach impoverished kids in Appalachia. Paul admired his choice. He had no money, no free time, no chance for promotion, but he had his students. *They need me Dad and I need them.*

"He does, but he took some time off."

"For what?"

"For you."

"For me?"

"Yes. We talked about this. We can't ignore the calendar. You don't have long and he wants to spend time with you. His students can wait, you can't."

Mary was referring to the talk she and Paul had, after the Doctor said he could do no more and that it would be a wise decision to return home, to spend the last few days with family and friends in a comfortable, familiar place. When they asked him how long, he had said, *Not long, but can't say for sure. A week, maybe two. I've even seen people hang on for months. Unlikely, but it's happened.*

Paul and Mary had agreed home was right and that they would cherish every day, whether it was one or 60. They identified Paul's closest living friends and family and made a list of names and decided it would be an invitation list. They contacted everyone on the list and invited them to say *Goodbye.*

"Randy was on the list. He's your son. He wants to see you."

"I understand. But, taking time off of work and flying in from Kentucky makes it all seem so immediate. I thought he'd wait a few weeks."

"Maybe he'll make two trips. One now, one in two weeks and if you're still around, maybe another next month."

"Three trips?"

"I'm sure he'd be happy to make three and many more."

Paul worried about his arrival. He'd flown to Minneapolis many times over the last 12-years. Paul had always met him at the airport. "How's he getting home?"

"Aly is picking him up. They'll be here by noon."

"Do I need to dress up, wear my new suit?"

"Nope. Pajamas and a sheet. That's it."

Paul knew. He'd never again be asked to choose between loafers and wingtips, pinstripes and solids, wool and cotton, blue and white. His closet door was closed, but he knew what was behind the door. His suits, his shirts, his pants, ties, belts and shoes, his work uniforms, costumes he used to hide his fear of judges and juries. It was all behind the door, pressed and polished, waiting to be worn. The wait would be long. Paul couldn't open the door and if he did, he had no need for the clothing that lurked there. He was in bed, in pajamas and would be, until he was no more.

"That'll be good. I miss Randy."

"And he misses you."

"Do you think their lives will change when I'm gone? Will my death change them?"

"You're their father. You were a good father. When you die, they'll cry, they'll grieve. They'll miss you. They won't be able to ask you a legal question or the name of the boy who played Harold in *Hazel*. When they're afraid, you won't be able to comfort them and when they need money, they can't call you. When you die, a part of them dies. It'll change them. It'll change me. It'll change Cliff, even Belle. You're a good man who's contributed a lot to a lot of people's lives. When you can no longer contribute, because you've moved on, others' lives will change. Most of all, your children's lives will change."

Mary was right. The *butterfly effect*. Every action has a reaction and so forth and so on. A misstep in January impacts the traffic in June. His absence would change things. It was inevitable, obdurate.

During his life, he had witnessed small morsels morph into lead laden agents of change. Minor brushes painted dark masterpieces and minor bumps derailed lives. Consequences. The aftermath of a word, a novel, the repercussion of a slight, suicide. Ramifications. *The butterfly effect.*

Paul met a classmate on a Main Street sidewalk in 1955 and they shared a cigarette and a story. Their exchange ended five minutes after it began, and Paul's friend stepped on his spent cigarette and off the curb, into the path of an oncoming Ford. Paul watched as his friend was pounded by the bumper, dropped by gravity and crushed by the heavy car's tires. He was dead before the smoke of his spent cigarette wafted into the atmosphere. It was traumatic to witness death, but what was more traumatic to Paul, was the realization that he had killed his friend. Not the car, not his friend's negligent, hazardous step, but Paul. If Paul had asked one more question, his friend would have delayed his step onto the pavement, would have avoided impact with the Ford and would still be alive. If Paul had asked his friend for a light or a cigarette, his friend would have delayed his step onto the pavement, would have avoided impact with the Ford and would still be alive. If Paul had delayed the punchline to the joke he told his friend, asked his friend why he wore tennis shoes instead of work boots, shook his friend's hand, looked down the road to see the fast approaching Ford or suggested his friend wait while traffic passed, his friend would have delayed his step onto the pavement, would have avoided impact with the Ford and would still be alive. Consequences. An obdurate, unanticipated consequence.

Paul felt responsible, recognizing his friend's sudden and unanticipated death resulted from an accumulation of happenstance and ever-moving variables that met on a road in Anoka, after two boys shared cigarettes and conversation. Paul could have changed the formula, upset the happenstance, altered the blueprint and rearranged the chairs, with something trivial, unimportant, and unnoticeable and his friend would have survived, perhaps to have married a woman who would have given birth to a child who would grow to formulate a product that would exponentially increase a seed's ability to bear fruit and end hunger in the world. Paul killed his friend and changed the world. Seeing his friend dead in the street, recognizing the impact he could have on others, that he could alter lives, mete consequences intentionally or unintentionally, adjust the future, Paul was frightened.

For years after Paul's friend died, Paul calculated his actions, moderating them so that they would have little impact on the world. He rarely drove, understanding if he did, his car would change traffic patterns and cause another Ford to rear-end a car sitting at a stop light, and kill an old lady driver. He stayed home from school when he felt a tickle in his throat, afraid that if he went to school, his bug would find a vulnerable host who would succumb to the virus and die. He shoveled his parent's sidewalk whenever a snow flake fell, believing if he didn't, an unsuspecting child would slip on ice covered concrete, strike his head on the unforgiving surface and join Paul's friend in the hereafter.

Paul's Dad wondered why his 17 year old son walked when he could drive, forfeited friends when he sniffled and shoveled the sidewalk when the snow began to fall, when it was falling and when it stopped. "What's wrong son?"

Paul explained his attempt to minimize his impact and spare the life of another. His Father listened intently and patiently and when Paul finished, his Father sat quietly and thought about what his son had said. Wise and loving, he emancipated Paul from his dread.

"What you say is true. What you do impacts others, often in ways that can't be anticipated. We're all inter-related, dependent on one another for direction. No question, if you get out there and do things, you'll change things, but what your theory fails to consider is, failing to act has equivalent impact on others as well. Three days ago, four people from Anoka were killed by a train when they crossed the tracks without looking. They died while you walked to the store and avoided your friends because you had a queasy stomach. If you had driven to the store, perhaps, your car would have met the car on a collision course with a train at an intersection and made it wait an extra-thirty-seconds. If you had, when the car approached the tracks, the place where it was crushed and its passengers died, the train would have been passing through the intersection and the soon to be dead driver would have seen it and avoided the collision."

It all seemed a bit too attenuated for the 17 year-old. Too many coincidences were needed before Paul could have saved the four lives. "Yeah, but what are the chances I would have slowed them down? A bit far-fetched."

"Absolutely. It's all far-fetched. But it's all possible. Before your friend died, would you have guessed that extending your conversation would have saved his life? Probably not." Paul confirmed his Father's suspicions with a shake of his head. "Right. That's the point. We can't predict all of the consequences of our actions. Or our inactions. We do things or don't do things and people die. We do things or don't do things and people live. Sometimes, our intentions are irrelevant. We can't control all of the consequences. But, if we know we will change the world, and we all do, the best thing we can do is, try to change it in a positive way. Make people happy. Make people smile. Shoulder the burden for others and hope for the best. If you're active, if you're trying to have a positive impact, you'll have impact, and likely the scorecard will reveal you made things better, not worse."

Paul thought about what his dad said and smiled.

Paul did as his Dad suggested. He tried to make things better, but sometimes he failed. In Vietnam, a Second Lieutenant asked

Paul to change duty days and when Paul did as his friend and fellow soldier suggested, his friend and fellow soldier was killed when on duty for Paul. He tried, and sometimes he succeeded. When Lauren was 15, she attended a party in the Cities and a friend's dad was to drive the kids home. Paul had represented the father and believed he had a problem with alcohol, so Paul insisted that he drive Lauren home. While he drove Lauren home, the other dad, with four kids in the car, was arrested for driving a motor vehicle while under the influence. Could someone have been hurt? Maybe, but Lauren was out of danger, because Paul decided to act.

He tried. Like everyone else, he changed the world, for better or worse. But he tried.

Paul pushed the button and the head of his bed rose, so that he could better look at Mary. "You're right. When I die, the kids will be changed, whether I want it or not. It's life, kismet, obdurate."

Mary wasn't satisfied with Paul's dismissive philosophy. She had heard the story of the Ford and Paul's friend, the boy who died while Paul watched, knew that he was focusing on unintended consequences when lamenting his legacy, questioning his impact. She knew better. "It's not just change for the sake of change. It's not *butterfly effect*. You were a good father. You helped raise three strong and happy kids. They all look like you, act like you and love you. You changed their diapers, their direction and their minds. You were almost always there, and they appreciated it then and they appreciate it now. They love you and will grieve when you leave. And why wouldn't they?"

"Because I'm old. Because I've been old for a long time. I haven't thrown a baseball to Randy in 30-years and it's been 25 years since I hit a tennis ball with Lauren. I danced with Aly when she was eight and at her wedding 15 years ago. I haven't been the Dad I was when they were young, for decades."

"So?" Mary didn't understand Paul's angst. Maybe it was death's doubt, a wistfulness created by knowing you've done all you can do, that time is running out. There wasn't much to add, time was an enemy.

"So? I wish I'd have danced more, tossed the ball more, hit more tennis balls as I got older. And now I can't. I can't be the dad I want to be."

"Obviously. I can't do the limbo or run a marathon. I got old. You did too. None of us can do what we were able to do when young. That's not the point."

"What is the point?" Paul was confronting maturity through dying eyes. Life was fair at 20, 30, 45, 60, 70, not so, at 75. A slip in speed? *Okay*. A little extra weight? *So be it*. Forget the names of people not important to you? *Fine*. But, not being able to walk to the bathroom or be able to relieve yourself without a catheter? *No way*. But, not being able to get behind the wheel and drive across town, to escape boredom and pick up your son at the airport? *Bullshit*. But, forgetting the name of your oldest grandchild because drugs combatting pain compromise memory? *Not acceptable. Bullshit*.

Mary hadn't heard Paul's silent debate, but answered the allegations as if she had. "The point is, when you could, you did.

When you can't, you can't. We've gotten old. We can't do it all anymore. It's called aging. aging. You adapt, the kids adapt. It's life. As you got older, your relationship with the kids matured. It's not any less than what it was, it's just different. The kids don't stop by to toss the ball, dance or hit tennis balls. They stop by to share their thoughts and to remember when you threw the ball, danced and hit tennis balls. It's different, but it's as good, as important."

Paul thought about what Mary said and smiled.

Mary had done what Paul's father had done fifty-years earlier. At 15, Paul was frozen, stuck, unable to move because he was afraid motion would leave casualties, and at 75, he was immobilized by side-rails and cancer, afraid immobility would diminish him as a parent and infect the memories of others. He didn't want them to forget the dad who threw a ball, served to his daughter on a tennis court or danced and beamed at a wedding. At 15 he was haunted by participation and at 75, he was haunted by his inability to participate. Paul's father rescued him at 15 and Mary rescued him at 75. With kind and wise words, they killed misperceptions and made it all right. Acknowledging that he tried and succeeded and that death wouldn't kill memories he created or the influence he had, he smiled. "You're right. It's tough to get old and even tougher to die."

Paul pushed the button and the head of his bed dropped. Mary checked the side rails, making sure they were up and locked in place, kissed Paul's forehead and said, "Get some sleep old man. It's not over yet."

chapter seven

Paul did what cancer patients on drugs do. He slept and he dreamed. His dreams, diced and morphed by opiates and an addled brain, were colorful, eventful. He danced on a tennis court and threw balls to his son. Mary was there, as was Lisa. They were friends, bonded by Paul. When Paul tired of dancing and throwing, he sat on a bench and Mary and the children joined him while Lisa walked away. Paul asked Mary why Lisa hadn't joined them on the bench and was told, *She can't be here, she doesn't belong.* When Lisa left the courts, when she disappeared, Paul heard sound bellowing from hidden speakers. Someone was testing the microphone and speakers. *Testing. Testing.* The voice was vaguely familiar, but he was unsure. *Dad?* And then Paul heard a clearly recognizable voice over the invisible public-address system. It was Lisa's voice, emanating from speakers hidden in the clouds. *See you soon.* When Paul looked to Mary to see if she had heard it, to determine if she understood it, she was gone. Paul was alone, on the bench, waiting. *Waiting for what?* And the bench changed to a bed, the sun to an overhead light and the fences surrounding the courts covered by windscreens, to siderails and the beige painted walls of Paul's bedroom. *Waiting for what?* "Dad? Good morning."

Randy stood over the bed and smiled at his father.

Woozy, under the influence of sleep and opiates, between sleep and awake and heaven and earth, Paul looked at his son and believed he was looking into a mirror warped by time. Same dark hair, same broad smile, same large nose with a bend to the right on the bridge, same clef in the chin and same small, brown, deep set eyes. If he grew his hair a bit and donned a blue, pin-striped suit, he could walk into the Supreme Court Courtroom and argue what Paul had argued 36 years earlier. Until he spoke, no one would notice the difference. Paul, 1976. Randy, 2015. Same man, different birthday.

As Paul's sleep-addled brain recovered from 14 hours of uninterrupted rest, Paul determined there was no mirror above his bed, that he wasn't gazing at himself, but his son. He coughed something from his lungs into his mouth, swallowed it, smiled and whispered, "Hi Randy. How are you?"

"Good. But my health isn't the issue. The question is, how do you feel?"

"Oh, I feel pretty good for a guy who will be dead in a few days."

Mary would have argued the point. Lauren and Aly would have as well. They would have attempted to buoy his spirits by invoking talk of miracles and unexpected delay. They would not have let Paul pronounce such a short timeline, without disagreement. *Don't say that. You never know. I read a Facebook post that said a stage IV cancer patient in hospice recovered, without medicine. A miracle they said. You never know. Don't give up.*

Not Randy. Honest. Straight shooter. Unable or unwilling to fib. The truth rode in his pant pocket and it didn't matter which pair of pants he wore or how many times they were washed, it was there, riding on a thigh, protected by cotton. Randy knew Paul was right and he wouldn't contradict him and upset what was in his pocket. "Well, if you're right, let's make it an incredible few days."

"How's Kentucky?"

"Challenging. Unlike anything I've ever known. A different world."

"In what way?"

"They have so little. Here, in Minnesota, no matter where in Minnesota, there are paved roads to take you to town, toilets you flush, doctors to care for the sick, food at the grocery store and clothing that fits and keeps you warm and dry. In the hills of Kentucky, the roads are rut filled and single lane, the toilets are in the woods and have no handle with which to flush, the sick remain sick until they recover without medical care or die, the food they eat is food they grew or killed with a bullet and the clothes they wear are the same clothes they wore last week or last month, clothes they wear until it no longer fits or the threads are so bare, it disappears. And they know nothing else. They were born without paved roads, indoor plumbing, grocery store food or medical care, and think that's just the way things are, the way things will always be."

"If it's so bad, why are you there? If things will never change, if you can't force change, why are you there?"

Paul knew the answer before he asked the question. Randy had told him when he decided to leave the law, and after his first year in Kentucky, when he returned home forlorn and pessimistic. Paul didn't disagree with his answer; he didn't ask the question again, because he wanted to challenge it or suggest a new and different answer, he asked because the answer he knew he'd receive made him proud of his son, confirmed he had done a good job as a father and that his son was a wonderful man. His cancer ravaged chest began to expand with pride before the answer was given.

"Because it's the right thing Dad. Because they need me. If I can help one kid escape, I'll be happy. If I can lift the burden, even a little bit, I'll be happy. Because it's the right thing Dad."

Paul smiled and his cancer filled chest swelled. "Good for you Randy. I wish I had just a little of your selflessness. It was always the money and the comforts that I chased. Your chase is so much more honorable."

"I got it from you, from Mom. You take no credit; you deserve credit. You took us to the State Fair when I was seven, and I don't remember the rides or the food, but I remember a young woman in tattered clothing with two dirty kids and you pulling out your wallet and giving her a twenty-dollar bill, when a twenty-dollar bill could last all day at the Fair. And I remember you tried to hide your generosity from us, blocking us from view of the gift giving and diverting our attention to the big, yellow slide. But, I saw it and I learned. Before you made that woman smile, you weren't enjoying the day. You were distracted, thinking about something other than the Fair, but after you shared with a stranger, your smile returned and you found joy in everything we did. You taught me that day, how important it is to give."

Paul remembered. He was surprised Randy had witnessed the exchange, money for a smile. Humble, Paul didn't want credit, didn't want his children to focus on the young family's poverty, so he hid his gesture, or at least, he thought he had. "It wasn't such a big thing. It certainly isn't equivalent with teaching in Appalachia."

Paul had never suffered. They always had what they needed and if they wanted to splurge, they did and the banker never knocked on the door in search of money. He had always defined generous as sacrificing, giving when there was little to give, being hungry because you fed the hungry with your only meal, tired, because instead of sleep, you gave your bed to those who needed sleep. Sacrifice. Pain. Longing. He had always had all he wanted, and as a result, didn't consider his gifts, acts of generosity. "My gift was convenient, easy to give. It wasn't like leaving a job that paid $150,000.00 for the hills of Kentucky and $22,000.00 annually."

"No. Probably not. But, I remember listening to you and Mom talk about your account receivables. So many people owed you money and when Mom asked, you said, *They can't afford to pay. It's okay, we have what we need.* When Lauren's high school team needed to rent indoor tennis courts and didn't have the money, you called the Tennis Center, paid for the courts and asked them to keep your gift a secret. And you have three kids who have college degrees, advanced degrees, and no debt. That wasn't magic. That was you and Mom. So, don't tell me you don't have my selflessness. I got it from you."

Paul's chest expanded again. He was dying, but as the lights flickered, with the help of an interpreter of his personal history, his son, who saw what he hadn't seen, Paul was proud of himself. *Good job old man.*

"Tell me about your Dad. I knew him, but only as my Grandfather, the guy who pulled an oxygen tank to the refrigerator to get a beer. He was slow when I knew him, unable to go for walks or toss a ball. He had a belly that was damn near as big as a wheel-barrow bucket and wobbly knees, but I don't know much about his days as a boy or young man. I've seen pictures of him and you, pictures before the belly, before wobbly knees, pictures of him smiling, wearing tennis shoes and shorts, so I know he was someone else way back then, but I don't know who. No books have been written about him, so you're the only source. When you're gone, he will be too, unless you share, so I can share and let him live in memories, forever."

Paul remembered. His Dad was a wonderful young man, an optimist whose positive outlook was buoyed by an American victory in World War II, an entrepreneur whose good fortune was crippled by mismanagement and progress. He smiled until he was forty-five and scowled to the grave, broken by failing health and an infected pocketbook.

"He was a good man. My earliest memories of him are from right after the War. He was a sailor, a Navy man. He called himself *Old Sea Dad*. I was born just before the War started, so your Grandmother got me through diapers and bottles alone, without help from your Grandpa. She was fighting infancy; he was fighting the Japanese. I remember going to the Union Depot in Downtown Minneapolis to greet him in 1945, after the War.

My mom, your grandmother didn't drive at that time, so her dad, your great-grandfather drove us to the Station. I remember that we parked blocks away from the Depot. There weren't parking places any closer. It was a carnival. Crowded. Everyone was happy, excited to see their personal heroes. The Depot was packed. It was hard to move. People everywhere. All excited, all happy. They were there, like we were, to meet someone who'd been away a long time, someone who survived the War."

"Were you excited?"

"That's complicated. Yes and no. I was filled with mixed emotions. For four years, I was the center of my Mom's universe. There was only me. When the War ended and she learned my Dad would be home soon, I wasn't quite so important. When she met friends for coffee, they didn't talk about baby rashes, colic, nighttime bed stories or playdates, they talked about their husbands, about their victory and impending return. Their smiles weren't any longer just for their kids, they were for their men. So, I kinda felt like my dad had relegated me to a secondary role. And, I didn't remember him and knew he'd be around soon and change my life. So, I was excited, the excitement was contagious, but I was also jealous and a bit apprehensive."

"And?"

Paul's memory of the reunion was clear. It was seared into his consciousness by its magic and impact. He remembered and he smiled, revealing teeth that hadn't been flossed in weeks, teeth that would never see a dentist again. Paul didn't care. It was 1945 and he was five years old.

"I was small, a weed amongst evergreens. I couldn't see beyond the butts of the people who stood between me and the platform that led to the train on which my dad was to arrive. When a large man stepped on my foot and I shrieked in pain, my Grandfather, your great-grandfather picked me up and held me high enough to protect my feet and see above the crowd.

"It was incredible. So many smiles, so many hugs, so many young men in uniform. There must've been a thousand discharged soldiers and sailors in the Depot, all relieved, all smiling, all looking for what they had left behind years ago. I didn't know what my dad looked like. He left before I was old enough to remember. We had pictures, but they were old, pictures of him as a child or new, pictures of him as a sailor, with a helmet pulled down over his eyes and masquerading the man. I scanned the crowd of heroes, but they all looked alike, tall, tan, erect, young and smiling.

"And then I saw him. Don't ask how I knew, I couldn't tell you then; I can't tell you now. He was a dot in a mass of veterans, the same size and color as the rest and 75 yards away, and yet, he was different than the rest, an island of color in an ocean of black and white. I saw and I knew; it was my Dad. And he saw me. Five-hundred stood between him and me, but he knew; I knew. His smile reached his earlobes and he walked to us. No, he walked to me. When he reached us, before he kissed my Mom, before he dropped his sea bag to the floor, he took me from my Grandfather's arms and hugged me. A minute? A lifetime? I was so happy, so proud. Jealousy disappeared; fear died. I was with my Dad."

Paul closed his eyes. He wasn't tired; he wasn't interested in sleep, he wanted to erase distractions of 2015, so he could see 1945 as it was then, as he wanted it to be now. Would he see his Dad in a few days? If so, would he be pulling an oxygen tank and sporting a watermelon above the belt-line, or would he be wearing his Navy Blues and hugging his son? *If he's wearing his Blues and hugging me, will I be five-years old? Good God, I don't know, but I'll soon find out.*

Randy was taking notes. The schoolteacher who taught Appalachians to write, wrote. He didn't want to forget.

"He'd given the Country four years of his life. Boys he graduated high school with, didn't survive. He was stationed on an island in the Pacific and his base was constantly strafed by Japanese planes. Friends died; friends survived. He limped, because a bullet from a Japanese plane struck a gas can, and when it exploded, shrapnel tore into his left calf. He used to tell war stories. They ended good or bad, some ending with injury or death, some ending with escape or enemy surrender, but he always said the same when the story was over. *Paul, war is scary, some men live and some men die, but those who live, men like me, live happily ever after, because they know two things, one that the world is a better place as a result of what they did, and two, they survived.*"

"Do you agree? You fought a war as well. Do you believe what your Dad believed?"

"Some of what he said is true for any war. Soldiers and sailors live and die, and those who survive, live life knowing that they are living on borrowed time. I have friends who died while standing near me, friends who died because they were where I should have been. They've been dead for nearly fifty-years, and here I am, with my family and friends. The last fifty have been a gift of survival. But, did we make the world a better place? I'm not sure. I don't think so."

Paul remembered a classmate who died in Vietnam. Art Dehn. A good guy. A kid. Art died when a sniper in a tree shot him dead. He remembered a black kid from New Jersey who sat on a mogul on a hill overlooking a bamboo swamp north of Da Nang, cleaning his rifle, a rifle he thought was empty, but wasn't and when the live ammunition fired, he was a dead black kid from New Jersey, lying on a mogul on a hill, overlooking a bamboo swamp. He remembered many who hadn't survived and wondered, *Are they waiting for me?*

"Did Grandpa's philosophy about war change?" Randy sat on a bedside chair, rested his notebook on his right thigh, put his pen on the paper and waited.

"No. The War was always a source of prideful memories for him."

"When did he change? The man I knew was not a robust, happy veteran."

"No, the man you knew was not the man I met at the Depot. The man you knew was different, changed, broken."

"How?"

"He got old. The habit that's killing me, ended his youth and killed his optimism. He learned to smoke in the Navy. They believed it would calm a sailor's nerves, so they promoted tobacco use. Gave the cigarettes away. He returned from the War smoking three packs of Camels a day. When he was 53, he had a heart-attack. The doctors said it was smoking that attacked his ticker. When he recovered, he was always tired, always short of breath, always anxiously awaiting the next heart attack. And he didn't have to wait long. Still smoking, two years later, at 55, he had another. They said he was lucky to have survived. I'm not so sure he agreed."

Randy raised his hand like a traffic cop, asking Paul to stop while he wrote. When he finished his scrawls, he dropped his hand and Paul continued.

"He began using oxygen and gaining weight. He drank to forget his plight, but the alcohol didn't help. He couldn't forget. When he stood and the oxygen tank tubes pulled at his nose, he remembered. When he gasped for air when doing something he had been able to do without effort for 50 years, he remembered. He couldn't forget."

Randy turned a couple of pages and read what he had written a half-an-hour earlier. "What about the business? You said something about being an unsuccessful entrepreneur."

"He was a good businessman. He had foresight. When he was discharged from the Navy, he considered his options. He was smart enough for college, but wasn't interested in delay. He wanted to get started. So, he decided to skip college and decided that he wanted to own a business, be his own boss. He did some research and learned that over-the-road trucks were displacing the railroads as the means of transporting goods cross-country. He had friends who had used veterans' benefits to buy large rigs and used them to haul goods across the country. He didn't want to go on the road for days at a time and miss his family, but wanted to take advantage of trucking, so he bought a parcel of land in Anoka, on U.S. Highway 10, a road that traveled from the east coast to the west coast, and built a restaurant for truckers. He sold food and gas. It was an immediate success. The parking lot was jammed with 16-wheelers and cars driven by his friends from Anoka, fellow veterans who had started their own businesses, grocery stores, shoe stores, television repair shops, gas stations, carpet stores, insurance agencies and small construction companies. He was a huge success. We lived in a nice house, drove nice cars, ate steak on Saturday nights and each Christmas, had a big tree surrounded by big presents. He was a huge success."

When Randy lowered his hand again, signaling that Paul could continue, he directed the conversation. "What happened?"

"Interstate 94."

"Huh?"

"While my Dad was recovering from his first heart attack, Interstate 94, a four-lane highway without traffic lights and the need to slow down for small towns, was being constructed. He was distracted, so didn't anticipate the changes the freeway five miles from his truck-stop would bring. The new highway opened at the same time as my Dad's second heart attack, and it was almost as deadly as the clots in his ticker. Immediately, truck traffic moved from 10 to 94, and when it did, my Dad's business died. A heart attack almost killed him and road improvements killed his business. And that's when you knew him. He was broken, physically and financially. The optimistic young war hero was a shadow, a memory, a has been. It was sad."

"And Grandma?"

"She was like other women of her day. She waited. While Dad fought the War, she waited for his return. When his business was new, she waited for it to succeed and when he was dying, she waited for him to die. She was always there, always supportive, always waiting. For what, I don't know. Most of the women of her day just waited, in the background, in a corner, under the covers. Waiting. And when he died, she began waiting to die. When she was sick, when it was clear she would soon die, when she was like me, imprisoned in her bed, I asked her how she felt, and she said, *I'm fine, I'm just waiting to see your Dad.*"

Paul believed it was a direct quote and important one. It summarized his Mother's life in nine words. He wanted Randy to get it right. He waited until Randy stopped writing and said it again, slowly, enunciating clearly, allowing Randy to read as he spoke. *I'm fine, I'm just waiting to see your Dad.*

Paul's travels to 1945 and 1970, tired him. He didn't want the conversation to end. He wanted to tell Randy how good it felt to catch a baseball in his glove, when it was thrown by his son. He wanted to apologize for his inattentiveness during Randy's first year and tell him that law was not as rewarding as a smile from a child. He wanted to tell him how proud he was. He had so much more to say, but didn't have the strength to say it. He hoped he had the time. As his eyelids drooped, Belle walked into the room, checked the I.V., noticed Paul's fatigue and said to Randy, "Let's let him sleep." She looked at her watch and continued. "I need to fortify the I.V. in about an hour-and-a-half, so I'm guessing, he'll sleep for a short nap and will be ready to share more memories in about an hour."

Paul smiled. Randy smiled. Belle smiled and Paul slept.

chapter eight

*P*aul exceeded expectations. Belle predicted 60 minutes of sleep; he woke 40 minutes after he closed his eyes. He rang the bell that rested on the tray at the side of his bed, and before the sound died, Randy stood in the open doorway. When he saw his father smile, he knew he rang not in distress, but rather in search of a companion. Randy was happy to be that companion and walked to the chair he earlier occupied and sat.

While Paul napped, Randy prepared for their conversation. *There's not much time left, I don't want to waste it wondering what to ask. Be productive, be prepared.*

"What do you think is the most significant change you've seen in your life?"

Perplexed, Paul furrowed his brow and looked at his son. "What, are you Morley Safer? *Most significant change?* I don't know what you mean. Thirty-nine years ago, you were floating in amniotic fluid in your Mother's belly and now you teach in Kentucky. That's pretty significant."

"That's not what I meant. In the world. What's the most significant change that has occurred in the world during your lifetime? Something significant, something that affects everyone, not just you and your family."

Paul tabulated a list. There were so many. *High speed travel? Advancements in medicine? Television? Computers? Integration? Cynicism?*

"Lots of options. Probably computers."

"Why?"

"When I was a kid, if you wanted to know what the neighbor thought, you'd ask the neighbor. You'd stand five feet apart and talk about whatever you wanted to talk about. Because you didn't want to offend the person who smiled at you when you said *Hello*, because you didn't want them to haul off and hit you if you said something offensive, your remarks were couched in soft, acceptable language. People worked hard to be civil, to get along. If something happened in the world or down the block, you waited until the newspaper hit the doorstep or the guy across the street knocked on the door, to find out. Now, you know what happened the minute after it happened and you communicate with your neighbor over the internet. You're not looking at a friendly face, you're not concerned about getting slugged, so you say what you want to say, without filters. Everyone's an expert, everyone's a critic. We don't try to forge alliances or maintain friendships. We don't discuss things civilly, we shout at our opponents after calling them boneheads, idiots, fuck-sticks or imbeciles. Computers have encouraged an impersonal world, a world where the person at the keyboard is right and everyone else is not only wrong, they're stupid, irredeemable."

Before he was confined to bed, Paul scanned Facebook and sometimes, added something to the discussion. After Donald Trump announced his candidacy, a classmate, a person Paul remembered with fondness, someone he hadn't seen in more than 50 years, someone Paul secretly desired when in high school, a blonde woman who played flute in the marching band, wrote that she was glad to see someone enter the presidential race who was unencumbered by political history.

After reading his classmate's post, Paul wrote, *Was surprised and happy to see you here. It's been a long time. Hope you're happy and healthy. Although I agree that Trump may be free from political baggage, he may be haunted by other baggage. Hope not, but think it's possible his personal and business history may create problems. Take care.*

Five minutes after hitting *Enter* and revealing his entry for everyone to read, the formerly diminutive flutist wrote, *Its hard for me to believe that someone who received the same education as me, could be so blind. You had always struck me as open-minded and bright. Guess I was wrong. The long Obama nightmare is nearing an end and hope you survive in your ignorance long enough to see how wrong you snowflakes have been.*

When Paul finished reading, his face flushed and his heartbeat quickened. *What? What? Unbelievable. Fifty plus years of fond memories destroyed in fifty seconds.*

Paul tried to mend the fence she constructed, with humor. *We did receive the same education, and I was taught that when its is used as a contraction for it is, it is spelled it's. Whatever. Hope there are no hard feelings. We just happen to disagree.*

Ten minutes after posting his unartful apology, without a melodic response from the marching-band flutist, Paul decided obtuse was the wrong tact, so decided to be more direct. He typed and sent, *Sorry if I offended you. It wasn't my intent.* Two seconds after Paul hit *Enter*, Facebook told him his message had not been posted and that he was no longer able to communicate with the woman who played flute and supported Don Trump. He had been blocked by once-upon-a-time bandmate.

The day his doctor discovered cancer in Paul's lungs, Paul told his Facebook friends he was sick. While waiting to read responses to his sad news, he scrolled down the page and read a post written below a picture of 12 white, middle-aged men who posed for the camera while holding semi-automatic rifles and wearing belts of bullets. The caption read, *Those who oppose the candidacy of Donald Trump, will answer to these great Patriots.*

Paul was focused on his health, his battle to restore good health and the creeping realization that perhaps it could not be restored, but when he read the *Patriots'* post, he reacted involuntarily. He was a lawyer who believed in procedures established hundreds of years earlier, and was offended by the apparent intimidation advanced by old white guys with guns and bullets. They seemed to say, *If he doesn't win, you're responsible and we'll use these guns and bullets to fix things, to forcibly impose what the system denied.*

Paul was offended by the short-sighted aggressive volley. He inhaled, exhaled, his heartbeat, once, twice…, his pupils narrowed as the sun entered the room, his brain relayed itch stimuli to his rash infested chest and he scratched, and he wrote. It was without contemplation. The words posted weren't mapped, considered or constructed. Like a beat of his heart or a breath by his lungs, he wrote. *If he loses because the people exercising rights given them by the Founding Fathers determine he should lose and you are unwilling to peacefully accept that, you are suggesting an insurrection and are no more patriotic than a Hitler sympathizer in 1940.*

Paul blocked the Patriots after receiving 24 messages in the three minutes following his response. *We know where you are, you're on the list. Did you see what we were holding in our trigger-happy hands? Snowflakes melt in the heat, we're the Son. Pussy. Get on board or get run over, asshole.*

Paul opened his eyes and looked at his son. His notebook was in his lap, his pencil silent. He was young, yet old school. He wasn't entering his words on a laptop or electronic tablet, he used paper and a pen. Left-handed, Randy smeared his words as he wrote, but he didn't care. Soap would remove the ink from the heal of his hand and the words he left on paper could be read, even though the letters weren't crisp and smear-free. He could put a plastic cap over the pen's ink tip and fold the paper littered with words and put it in his pocket and carry it to the bathroom, a restaurant or his grave. Old school. He made it, could hold it and could carry it to where he wanted to carry it. Old school. He smiled and his Dad continued.

"I'm afraid we don't like each other much anymore. The computer and internet communications have insulated us from others and immunized us from civility. We don't get along and many have no interest in doing so. Arrogance. Egoism. Insensitivity. Myopic reasoning which dismisses others and leaves no room for compromise. We're at each other's throats and don't seem to care. With 350 million Americans and seven billion people, all pulling in different directions, all trying to do what's personally best for him or her, without consideration for others, the future's not bright. And from my perspective, it's all brought to you by the age of computers."

"But Dad, computers help us share information and disseminate data to find solutions to the World's problems. The internet may have some dilatory affect, but computers on the whole, are helpful."

"You're right, computers can be helpful. Without computers, we'd not be able to analyze DNA or find the right combinations to combat cancer or AIDS, but if computers continue to isolate and insulate us, hate will prevail and neither good health nor prosperity will be adequate compensation."

"Really? You believe that?"

"I do. I fear that. Trump may be elected. A complete moron. An egocentric, selfish puke. He pedals hate on the internet and it's working. Divide and conquer. He calls Mexicans rapists and murderers, President Obama an illegal born in Kenya and reporters who question his ability, unworthy peddlers of fake news.

Without the internet, that guy is nothing more than a blowhard with a misshapen head and crop of coiffed golden retriever fur. With it, he's a credible candidate. That's scary."

"I'm not so sure. He'll drop out before he gets elected. He loves the attention. He doesn't want to be president."

"I hope you're right, but it makes little difference. We're posed to elect a Trump. If not him, someone like him, someone who feeds the discord. If not that prick, another, similar prick."

Randy put his pen in his pant pocket. This was not a conversation for posterity; this was conversation between men with different opinions. Paul's health was irrelevant. It wasn't a *he's soon to be dead conversation,* it was just talk between two men. "But, we've made changes in the past to secure a healthy future and I think we will again. Too much gloom and doom from your perspective."

"When I'm added to a list by gun toting clowns who consider themselves patriots and am blocked by a woman who broke my heart more than fifty years ago, both for sharing a belief, the gloom and doom appears."

"It'll get better. Wait and see. People want to connect. It's our nature. We want others to like us and when they don't, we feel bad. The internet is relatively new. It'll get old, and when it does, we'll shut down the laptop and cross the street to talk face-to-face with our neighbors. It's inevitable. Wait and see."

"I can't."

"You can't what?"

"Wait and see. I'll be dead before it changes. Your future is decades long, mine is days long. Change may be inevitable, but it happens slowly. Things may get better, but I won't live to see it."

"Sorry. I forgot."

Paul smiled. He was glad that Randy forgot. There were times Paul forgot. When he responded to the *Patriots* intimidating post, when he told Mary that *Doctor Zhivago* was really, really long when marijuana interfered with his internal clock, when he told Randy that his Grandfather had been a nice and loving man, capable of smiling and succeeding in business, before ill health and progress derailed him, he forgot that he was dying and remembered, unclouded by his impending demise. He was better able to live when he was not lacquered in death. "No need to apologize. I forget sometimes too. It's a good thing. Focus on living, not dying. It's a good thing."

"But, I don't want you to die believing all is lost. We have problems. Maybe Trump will be elected, but we'll survive Trump. We survived the Great War, the Depression, World War II, the Cold War, four Super Bowl losses, Lincoln's assassination and disco. We'll survive Trump and the internet."

"You're probably right. I think I react to what I've seen and if I can't see a time when I benefit from the positive changes, I conclude they'll never happen. For your sake, I hope they do, and your opinion on the future is much more important than mine. You can change it, I can't. I won't be here."

Randy disagreed. Even though his Dad would be burned and his ashes scattered in downtown Anoka, he believed he'd still be there, still changing things.

"Tell Lauren, Alyson and their kids that you'll have no impact on the world after you're dead, and I promise you, you'll get an argument. You made us and helped form us. What we do, we do, in part because of you. Your influence will live long after you're dead. If Trump is elected, will I sit idly by and let him destroy us? No. Why? Because I'm your son, because you taught me the difference between right and wrong and that good people oppose the bad. And if the internet promotes anger, division and hate, Lauren will do everything she can to moderate its influence and promote unity and love. And when corporations choose profits over the environment, your grandkids, taught by you and your kids, will stand tall and say *No more*. You'll be dead, but you'll live on."

Paul knew Randy was right. He didn't need more proof to accept the proposition. He'd be here after he wasn't, and he knew it. It was what Mary had said not long ago. He was convinced. *I'll live forever*. Paul needed no further proof, but he asked for it anyway, recognizing the offer Randy would soon provide, would make him happy, help him forget that his bed had side-rails, locked to keep the sick in bed.

"Are you sure?"

"Absolutely. Remember, I teach in Kentucky, because you gave a poor woman twenty dollars to enjoy the fair. Parents were better able to pay for their children's educations, because you didn't demand that they pay you for your time. Soldiers with whom you served in Vietnam, survived because you were there and they now have children who search for the cure to cancer or have raised children who will oppose Trump or a Trump-wanna-be. If a man raises his hand to one of your daughters' she will defend herself, because you taught us all that violence between a man and a woman is always wrong and should never be tolerated. And good people who learned lessons you taught, are teaching others what they discovered through you. You can die old man, but your death won't diminish your impact. We're not amnesiac. We won't forget. You'll live on."

Paul was glad he had decided to delay death and temper it with medicine; he was pleased he had decided to die at home. When the doctor told him, he was going to die, Paul reacted instinctively, naturally. He forgot about the 75 years of life well lived, and focused on the 75 days remaining, the days that presumably led to a painful death. It was hard; it was almost over, and he didn't want to leave. He wanted the Doctor to amend his diagnosis, to tell him it was all a mistake. He wanted to slip into a rabbit's hole and emerge, youthful, healthy. He dreaded the remaining days and was haunted by denial and lambasted by fantasy. He was miserable, afraid of the darkness. When he gave up, when he accepted there was nothing more to do, when he decided to combat pain with pills and let life end on its terms, he was given an opportunity to live. The time was short, but it was his time, unfettered by dread, pain and regret. And, the time was devoted to smiling and memories, happy ones, memories that reminded Paul it had all been worthwhile.

"Thanks Randy."

"For what?"

"For everything. You make me proud, of you and quite frankly, of myself. Thanks."

Paul considered another nap. His energy was depleted, it almost always was. He'd rest, for an hour or 13, consume calories digging himself from sleep's abyss, and when he emerged, there was only enough for a short visit, a modest return to yesterday when smiles were evident, the future bright and time abundant. He was tired, but uncertain how long he'd be away if he closed his eyes. It could be minutes, hours or forever. He was unwilling to risk it.

"Remember when you and Tom Darcy camped on the Rum River?"

"I do. We were about 12 and thought we'd slay a deer with our jackknives and roast it over a campfire. We pitched a tent on the Boy Scout Campground, about two miles out of town in July, and even though you were to pick us up the next morning, Tom and I thought that we'd need a strategy to combat the upcoming cold winter. And before it was dark, we regretted our decision to camp. Neither of us slept. We heard the trees rustle in the wind and imagined an evil animal crawling on branches above our tent. We heard small nocturnal animals cross fallen, dry leaves and imagined hungry, flesh-eating bears planning an attack. The sun was below the horizon for only eight hours, but we counted every minute and it seemed like days. Yeah, I remember."

"Me too. While you two exercised your independence, I worried about the same things you worried about, bears, coyotes, trees bending and breaking in the wind, boys too curious to remain in their tent, boys who explored in the dark and waded into fast currents and were then, unable to see the shore. You didn't sleep. Neither did I. Growing older is hard on everyone, including boys and dads."

"And I remembered when you got there, to pick us up, Tom and I argued with you, tried to convince you to let us stay one more night. Thank God you said *No*. If you'd have said *Yes*, I don't know what we'd have done. We couldn't have survived another night."

"So many dances." As they waltzed across the floor of life, Paul led, but allowed his dance partners, his children, an opportunity change the step, the pace, the experience. It had been Paul's nature, to worry about his kids, yet his conscious decision, to hide his concern. His Mom was a worrier and she did nothing to hide it. If Paul left the house to walk down the block to the grocery store, she cautioned, *Cross only at the intersection and please, don't get hit by a car; I couldn't take it.* If he told her he was going to fish at the end of the dock, she'd warn him of the perils. *Don't go in the water, it's deep and cold and if you lean over the edge of the dock to look into the water, make sure you keep your weight back, over the dock, because if you don't, gravity will pull you into the water and if you drown, I couldn't take it.* When he learned to drive, when he opened the door to leave the house and rattled his car keys for his Mom to see, she warned, *Go slow, watch the traffic, be observant, of pedestrians and other cars, keep your radio off and avoid other distractions and please don't get in an accident, especially a serious one where you or someone else is injured, I just couldn't take it.*

His Mother's worries had henpecked Paul. As a child, he rarely took chances, always calculated the risks and always looked both ways before crossing the road, asking a girl on a date, ordering from the menu or choosing the clothes to be worn for the day. He ignored deviations and was allergic to spontaneity. He was much too cautious and wanted more for his kids, so even though he inherited his Mother's fearful proclivities, he shielded his children from them. He fretted rather than caution and laid awake rather than impinge on his children's ability to take a chance. Now, it was too late and confession instructive, not harmful.

"You know I always worried about you kids. I always thought that danger lurked just around every corner. I got that from my Mom. And she let me know she worried, and so, I learned to worry and rarely took chances in my life. I wanted you guys to take chances, so I never let you know I worried."

"I knew. You didn't hide it from me. You were always awake when I came home, no matter how late. When I asked for permission, you typically said *Yes*, but you always took the time to consider your options and the riskier the experience, the less blood there was in your face when you said *Yes*. And you didn't let Tom and I camp out for one more night. I knew."

"I was raised in a worrier's home and that made me a worrier. And when you get older, you've had enough experience with danger and damage to know it's there and can find the unsuspecting. I've been bitten by unfamiliar dogs; I was in a car accident; I've been punched by a jerk, changed a flat tire on a freeway and have been out of money in the cold, without gasoline or a weather tested battery to start my old and stiff car. I didn't want you kids to combat those same problems, but on the other hand, I understand, because I had all of those experiences, I can confront almost anything."

"Well, I've never been punched or been bitten by a scared dog, but I did survive a night in the woods, haunted by tree dwellers and hungry bears. You gave me opportunity to suffer and learn. Thanks for the lesson."

Before he could congratulate himself for being a good father, Belle walked in the room and smiling, asked Randy to leave. She adjusted Paul's I.V., injected it with opiates and changed the diaper Paul wore. After disinfecting him with wipes, drying him with powder and closing the diaper with Velcro tabs, Belle asked, "Anything I can do?"

"Don't do as the last person who changed my diapers did, make me worry."

Belle smiled. There was little else to worry about at this stage. Money? Irrelevant. Employment? Irrelevant. Fertility? Irrelevant. Popularity? Irrelevant. Good health? Unattainable and irrelevant. "Don't worry, be happy."

"Thanks, I'll try. Send Randy in please."

Belle nodded her head, did as asked, but before Randy returned, Paul's eyes were closed and he slept. He dreamed. He was on the banks of a river. Heavy creatures howled in the trees above and large, plodding beasts circled their camp, but Paul was unafraid; there was nothing left to lose and Randy was there, protecting him from the unknown with a jackknife, a smile and confidence grown in experience. *Don't worry Dad. I'm here.*

chapter nine

*W*hile Paul slept, the sun disappeared and appeared again, the air conditioner cycled on and off 14 times, Donald Trump appeared at two campaign events, mocked a disabled journalist and denied he ever called a woman a pig, *except for Rosie O'Donnell.* The 10 o'clock news was all Trump. His detractors laughed at his amateurism, while his supporters defended him against unprecedented scrutiny and proudly proclaimed, *He's not a politician.* While Trump campaigned for the presidency by criticizing the opposition, and ridiculing them for imperfections, Paul slept in shades of blue, garnished with memories from the old neighborhood, when Anoka had no stop lights and few stop signs, when veterans from the Spanish-American War and World War I walked in parades on Memorial Day and the Fourth of July, when church bells signaled five o'clock and children played, without supervision or fear. Two dreams, Trump's and Paul's, one a nightmare the other a graceful glide to death.

When Paul woke and opened his eyes, allowing the fog to escape, he saw Alyson, Lauren, Randy and Mary at the end of his bed, while Belle adjusted the bag that dripped the magic elixir into his blood. Knowing the Doctor had suggested Paul visit with only one person at a time, that a visit with too many could cause stress and death, Paul asked the question he formulated when he discovered his entire family in his room. "Am I dead?"

Alyson was always ready, always coiled tightly and waiting to be sprung. Her teachers called her disruptive, her classmates called her impatient, her parents called her eager. She couldn't wait. If it had to be done, she did it as soon as she learned what needed to be done. She was so determined to get to it, she sometimes forgot what she was getting to. Lauren was a runner, Randy, a walker, Alyson, a pouncer. Always ready, always enthusiastic, always anticipating, always smiling, always naively honest.

"We didn't know Dad. You slept for 12 hours and we weren't certain. If you didn't open your eyes and your heart stopped, we all wanted to be here. You know. The obits always say, *Passed to the other side with his family by his side*. We want to be honest when we write it and have no interest in writing, *Passed to the other side with his family, except for Randy and Alyson, by his side*. But, I for one, am glad you opened your eyes and then your mouth and spoke. I'd rather talk to you than take pride in our honesty when reading your obituary."

Paul wasn't sure he'd heard right. He'd always had a hard time understanding what his youngest said. She was loud enough, but the words came out of her mouth like popcorn cooking on a hot stove, sometimes two at a time, sometimes three at a time. She was in such a hurry to say the fourth word, she sometimes said it over the third and on occasion, before the third. Most would have taken 30 seconds to say what Alyson said; it took her 13 seconds. "Huh?"

Mary took the time necessary to explain. "We weren't sure this was the time and all wanted to be here if it was."

Paul smiled at his impatient, impetuous, sweet, small girl and said, "That's what I thought she said."

Belle completed her task, walked to the foot of the bed so she stood with the others and said, "Well, now that we've got *that* clear, let's leave him alone with Alyson. Ok?"

All but Alyson nodded their heads and turned to follow Belle out the door. Before the four had passed the threshold, Alyson had asked three questions and made a simple statement. "How do you feel Dad? Can I get you anything? I didn't offend you, did I? If I did, I'm sorry."

Paul smiled. She was always a challenge, but so damn cute, sincere and well-intentioned. She had always acted as if she were the one condemned to die soon. It was as if a premonition warned her, told her to get it done while she could, that there was little time and absolutely no time for contemplation. "I'm fine. I don't need anything and wasn't offended. I'm dying, the question is *When?* I ask it all the time. Every time I close my eyes, I wonder if I'll open them again, so you didn't say anything I haven't already said to myself."

"Good. Not good that you think those things too. I didn't mean I'm glad you wonder if you you'll wake after sleep. It's not what

I meant. Not at all. Hope it didn't sound like that. I just meant, it's good that I didn't offend you."

"I understand Aly. That's what I thought you meant. No offense taken."

It had always been this way. Alyson was unrelentingly kind to an imperfection. She was sensitive and wanted nothing more than to please everyone, people she knew, people she didn't know, people she liked, people she didn't like, everyone. In sixth grade, she was elected her elementary school queen. First through sixth grade students voted for one of three candidates, each chosen by her sixth-grade class, and the victor was crowned Queen, and rode in a convertible emblazoned with a sign that read, *WASH-INGTON ELEMENTARY QUEEN*, in the Halloween parade. Aly won because she was kind, friendly, enthusiastic and fun. She wanted everyone to like her, and she succeeded.

When Aly learned that a competitor, another girl from sixth-grade, the nominee of another class, was devastated by the results of the election, that she had cried for days and likely needed the Queen's crown to combat low self-esteem, Aly tried to abdicate her throne. "I don't want to be Queen. Give it to Angela. She's much more deserving."

Aly's Principal wasn't persuaded. "But, Alyson, the students elected you to be their queen. We can't ignore the vote."

A recount? A stomachache on Halloween? Abdication? The evening before she made her plea to her principal, she and Paul had discussed her options. Paul was proud of her willingness to forfeit adulation for another's feelings. He used the word *abdication*, and after explaining it to Aly, heard her use it a dozen times, at dinner, bedtime and the breakfast table.

The Principal was not easily convinced. "It's not that easy, Alyson."

"King Edward abdicated his throne to marry an American. He said it and it was done. It's not that hard Principal Cooper."

And so, on Halloween in 1990, Alyson stood on the curb without a stomachache, and waved at Angela Morton, who rode in a convertible emblazoned with *WASHINGTON ELEMENTARY QUEEN*, and smiled.

"Dad, are you scared?"

"A little. It's almost over, and I don't know for certain, where I'll be in a week or two. It's kinda frightening."

"Oh, I know where you'll be. You'll be in the best place possible. No one is more deserving than you. I'll miss you, I already do, but, I'm not afraid for you. You'll be just fine. No question. Just fine."

"Thanks Aly."

Aly held her father's hand. Even though she had lots to say and it took all of her strength to not say it, she said nothing. She knew she was a handful, hopefully a pleasant handful, but knew her Dad needed peace, quiet and rest, something she was, by nature, typically unable to give. She fought her nature and said nothing.

"Aly, do you remember Angela Morton?"

"Yes, I do."

"That was a good thing you did for her. I was proud. Still am."

"Lot of good it did."

Angela committed suicide in ninth grade after her boyfriend moved on to another.

"It did a lot of good. Angela was obviously depressed. If not, the election loss wouldn't have made her cry for two days and her boyfriend's escape wouldn't have caused her to kill herself. She probably didn't have many happy days, depression saw to that, but one happy day she had, was on Halloween in 1990. And you, young lady, gave her that happy day."

"Thanks Dad. I wish I could have given her more. I wish I could have helped her beat her demons."

"We all wish that Sweetheart, but some things you can do and some things you can't. You did what you could, more than many would have, and because of what you did, Angela had a happy and blissful ride in a convertible."

"Do you think Angela liked me Dad?"

"I don't know Honey. I didn't know Angela. But, I can't understand why she wouldn't have liked you."

"I liked her. She was withdrawn and didn't say much, but, I liked her."

"You like everyone. I wish I was more like you."

"Well, if you're not, you hide it well. I've heard you grumble about people to Mom, but have never heard you criticize someone in public. I've never seen you do something that hurt anyone."

"For you, it's natural. You're kind by nature, maybe too kind. Me, I have to fight it. I bite my tongue and try to do the right thing. But, it's not natural."

"I don't remember you making someone feel bad."

"Pete Talbot?"

"Well, that couldn't be avoided."

It could have been, but it wasn't. Paul and Pete attended law school together and after both worked for the government and large law firms, they formed a partnership. *Thomas and Talbot.* Pete and Paul were partners and very good friends. They worked together, dubbed the golf ball around the golf course together, ate lunch together, had a beer after work together and socialized with their families, together, during the weekends.

Five years after the partnership was formed, Paul determined it should be dissolved. Paul wasn't materialistic, didn't care about money, so long as he had enough to pay the bills, sock some away for retirement and the kids' college educations and make the occasional spontaneous, unnecessary, irresponsible, fun purchase, but when he looked at the Firm's books, he learned that he collected 80% of the fees and worked two-times as many hours as Pete, and that didn't sit well. They had conversations about effort and collections, but Pete never took the conversations seriously, often ending them with, *You knew what you were getting when we joined up my friend. Sorry.*

An associate at *Thomas and Talbot* started doing the work Pete had done when the Firm was formed and Pete was rarely seen in the office. When he appeared, he smiled, was boisterous and bold, told people what to do, dipped into petty cash and left. His arrivals and departures most often occurred when Paul was in court or at lunch, so Paul was unable to confront him when he was in his most vulnerable, obnoxious position.

They stopped golfing together, late afternoon rounds of beer at the Legion disappeared and joint family get-togethers were just distant memories. Paul sent Pete a letter, a letter he didn't want to sign, but a letter he needed to sign, that told Pete things needed to change or the partnership would be dissolved, but Pete didn't respond. Out of options, Paul brought Aly to the office, parked a block away and waited for Pete to appear, give orders and take cash. Pete was appropriately smitten with Aly. He called her the *Energizer Bunny* and lifted and twirled her every time they met. She was Paul's protector, his shield, his guarantee that Pete would accept the news without creating a scene. He wouldn't act childish in front of the *Energizer Bunny*.

Paul took the steel box that held petty cash, about a-thousand-dollars in currency, to his office, knowing Pete would need to see him if he wanted money. At 12:15, Pete knocked on Paul's office door, walked in, saw Aly on the floor with Legos and said, *"Energizer Bunny,* how are you?" After lifting Aly and twirling her high in the air, avoiding light fixtures and an overhead fan, Pete sat her down by her Legos and waited until she clamped one to another and searched for the perfect third. He looked at Paul, chose his words carefully and said, "Paul, I need some petty cash. Got to stop at the grocery store and didn't bring my wallet with me."

"Sorry Pete. No petty cash."

Pete wasn't surprised by what his partner said, likely he expected it. He smiled, looked at Aly who looked at Legos, returned his gaze to his partner, buttoned the second button from the collar, transforming himself from casual to business casual and continued. "I know I've been gone a lot and haven't contributed much lately, but that'll all change soon. And, the petty cash is as much mine as yours and I need some."

"Sorry Pete, it's over."

Pete unbuttoned the button he'd just buttoned, transforming himself from constrained to loose and unhindered, cleared his throat two times, interlocked his fingers, bringing praying hands to his chin and asked, "What do mean it's over?"

"It's over Pete. The partnership. It's over."

His prayer unanswered, Pete separated his hands, formed fists and asked for a different answer. "No. Can't be. We can work this out."

"Sorry my friend, I've tried for six months and you've ignored me. I've considered the options and concluded; the partnership needs to be dissolved. You're a great guy Pete, but you haven't been a good partner. Sorry my friend."

Pete spoke, more loudly, more accusatorily. Aly left the Legos and focused on the men. "Paul, I own one half of this place. You don't have the right to take it from me."

Pete was on his way to shouting, to defending, to accusing, but before he could lift his voice so that everyone on the block could hear, Aly spoke. She was frightened, surprised to see her Dad and the man who lifted and twirled her, have angry words. She didn't understand. "Daddy?"

Paul didn't answer his daughter with words. He looked at her and smiled. His smile was more articulate than words. Aly breathed a sigh of relief and sheepishly returned to her blocks.

Pete did as Paul expected. Aly, Paul's shield, his protector, his guarantee, inserted herself into the men's argument and diffused it. *Daddy?* It was enough. Pete looked at the *Energizer Bunny*, smiled, lowered his voice and asked, "Well, then, what do we do?"

"We divide everything equally. You're right, this is one-half yours and I have no desire to take it from you. So, we decide amongst ourselves how things are to be divided, clients, equipment, accounts receivable, the phone number, the office building and the staff, or we ask someone to help."

Pete wasn't pleased. He was surprised and shaken. He sat in a large leather chair in front of Paul's desk, hung his head and cried. He didn't sob, didn't snort, didn't audibly weep, but it was clear he cried. A tissue dabbed water from his eyes as his shoulders slumped and shook with each choppy breath he took.

Alyson stopped playing with blocks and walked to Paul and looked over the desk at Pete. "Daddy?"

Paul lifted Aly to his lap and waited in silence for Pete to regain composure. When Pete lifted his head, and looked at Paul with dry eyes, Paul offered condolences and hope. "It was a good run Pete. We'll do fine in separate shops. And hopefully, we can remain friends."

Paul offered Pete his hand, but Pete stood, looked at Aly and without shaking Paul's outstretched hand, said, "Alyson, be a good girl." He left the office.

Paul and Pete were able to divide *Thomas and Talbot* amicably, although Pete hired a lawyer who met with Paul and helped iron out the details. Paul rarely saw Pete after the separation and when he did, it was formal, cordial. Alyson saw Pete three times, once at a school play, once at a soccer game and once on the sidewalk in front of a window that read, *Pete Thomas Law Office*. Each time they met, Pete smiled, was inclined to lift and twirl, but didn't. He looked at the little girl, was tempted to say *How's the Energizer Bunny?*, but after digging deep to remember a name he never used, instead said, *Hello Alyson*.

"What happened to Pete Dad?"

"Last I heard, he lived in Florida and worked for H and R Block preparing taxes. But, I'm not sure. I kinda miss him."

"Me too. Do you remember what he called me?"

Paul did, but he wanted the memory refreshed by someone else. "No, what?"

"*Energizer Bunny.*"

"That's right. And do you know why?"

"No. I never thought about it. Why?"

"Because you and the original *Energizer Bunny* didn't stop. You both kept on ticking like a Timex watch."

"Me? I stop. When there's nothing left to say, I stop. When the job is done, I stop. When there's nowhere to go, I stop. Why would he think I never stopped? I'm always stopping. I love to have nothing more to say, nothing more to do. I'm happiest when I'm quiet and still. I don't understand."

Alyson reflected and smiled. Although there was much more she wanted to say, she said only one thing and left it at that. Short, to the point, so unlike Alyson. "I get it; I know."

Paul closed his eyes and opened them five minutes later. Alyson sat in the chair on the side of Paul's hospital bed, sipping coffee, eating a bagel, listening to music, reading a book and answering Facebook posts. *Only five things at once?* Paul smiled and announced his return. "I'm back."

"While you napped, I found Pete. I did a Google search on my tablet. I found his obituary. He died six years ago. In Florida. I know it was him, because the obituary mentioned Minnesota, listed his kids and identified his surviving spouse. It was him. Sorry Dad."

"That's okay. Maybe he'll greet me when I pass through. Will he be the responsible partner, the irresponsible one or a guy completing tax returns? Will he be who I want him to be, what he wants to be or something someone or something else wants him to be? That's the question. Do children who died in childbirth remain infants, unable to walk, read, talk or fend for themselves? Do people who die feeble, with non-existent memories, pass and need walkers and help with recollections in the hereafter? It's a mystery. I don't have the answer, but will soon enough. Too bad I can't share it with you when I learn."

"What would life be without mystery? I don't want to know. I'll keep searching, keep wondering, keep guessing, but quite frankly, I don't want to know. The search keeps us all going. If we know the answers to the most important questions, maybe we stop. I don't want to stop; I want to keep going, like an *Eveready Bunny*."

"You are my live-wire. Always have been. You're a doer. Always doing, always looking for the next thing to do."

"Which is why I teach kindergarten. Always something to do. They're young. Can't know it all by 3:30. Always something new to teach. It never ends. And, they like me. I landed right. Unending tasks to be done for the kids that surround me, the kids who like me, the kids who need me. Perfect."

Paul helped in Aly's classroom. She was impressive. She was the best educated, biggest, five year old in the room. She sat on the floor when the kids sat on the floor. When the kids and Aly formed a circle, she sat in a chair, the color and size as the chairs on which the children sat. If the children got excited about a project, the most excited person in the classroom was their teacher. She was enthusiastic, impatient, kind, eager. She was where she should be, in a classroom with hungry children.

A plodding conversation wasn't enough for Alyson. She needed more than an exchange of words with a dying man. He was her father and she wanted to be there, to share with him, but in between the sentences, when he reflected silently, when he contemplated his answer, she was lost and hungry for something else. She couldn't put earbuds in her ears and listen to music or open the pages of a good book; both would be rude, and entertain her exclusively, leaving her dad alone with his thoughts. "Want to watch television?"

It was noon. TV? Soaps and news. *The Capital Report* or *All My Children*. Trump or Erica Caine. A self-important character reading a script or a soap-opera actor. Aly was a people pleaser, in part, because she inherited the trait from Paul. Like her, he wanted to please everyone, especially his youngest, precious child and understood a dying man wasn't able to satiate her need for intellectual stimulation and fill the gaps she saw. He needed help; he couldn't do it alone. "Sure. T.V.'s good."

Aly reached for the closest remote control, pushed the big red button, and the head of Paul's bed began to lift. She dropped the devise to the table alongside the bed, searched for the television's remote control and apologized. "Sorry. I should slow down and read the instructions, or at least the button."

When the picture filled the screen, Paul saw a woman in her fifties, wearing grand earrings, perfectly applied makeup and an evening dress, while standing in a kitchen and wearing a sneer. Paul asked, "Erica Caine?"

"No. That show's off the air. Don't know who she is. Just one more."

Alyson scrolled through the channels looking for something of interest. She saw cops arresting a drunk man with a mullet, wearing cut-off blue jeans and a tee-shirt that read *I'm Not With Stupid, I'm Stupid*, a plump woman selling something designed to remove stubborn lids from slippery jars, a weather report from Nashville, three soap operas, a basketball game played in 1992, a baseball game played the day before, a self-proclaimed Christian absolving sins and asking for donations, *money for Christ*, six movies, all too long and slow to entertain a dying man and his soon-to-be-grieving daughter with an over-active mind, three cartoons and news. She asked Paul if he had a preference and when he indicated he did not, she stopped at CNN.

An attractive, business-like woman delivered the headlines. She was pleasant, but not too pleasant, appropriate given that she reported on death and misery. She was succinct, but not too succinct, given she needed to provide enough irrelevant, salacious bits of fodder to keep the audience interested. She was deferential to those to whom she spoke, interested to hear what they had to say, but not so deferential that her credibility as a professional journalist was compromised. She tip-toed a winding and narrow road.

A family of four has been murdered in Houston and police have no evidence to explain why the crime was committed. Paul wondered if he'd meet the slain victims when he died and would soon learn what police did not know. *Interested in a new direction and hoping to steer Ted Cruz and Donald Trump supporters to his campaign, Wisconsin Governor Scott Walker contacted an experienced Republican operative and inquired about his willingness to join the Walker campaign.* As a supporter of unions, which Walker had offensively challenged in Wisconsin, Paul grinned at the Governor's inability to attract a following and concluded it wasn't about who was running the campaign, but rather the candidate. *The President of NBC News issued a statement today. "Due to the recent derogatory statements by Donald Trump regarding immigrants, NBCUniversal is ending its business relationship with Mr. Trump. At NBC, respect and dignity for all people are cornerstones of our values."* Paul smiled, agreed with the network and hoped the statement was a harbinger of bad things to come. *Prick.*

*It's hot in New York City. **Not here, not in my bedroom.** The glaciers in the Arctic are disappearing at an alarming rate according to the United States Environmental Protection Agency, and it predicts, unless something is done soon, the World will be beyond the tipping point in less than a generation. **Nothing more I can do, nothing it can do to me, but I fear for those who are young and will give birth to a generation who will battle floods, tornadoes, unrelenting heat and oxygen depleted*** *air. Opponents of gun control, frightened that President Obama will issue executive orders restricting their right to bear arms, marched on Washington.* **Too many guns make them available to everyone, including those who want to use them illegally.**

While the news program was in commercial break, Paul thought about what he had watched and how he had reacted. Every story told by the anchor, generated a visceral response. Paul listened, he heard, he internalized and he reacted. The stories were lost in the interpretation. Paul didn't care about the heat in New York City, because he wasn't hot in hospice. Paul didn't care about what scientists said about climate change, he recognized he was insulated and his offspring would shoulder the battle. It didn't matter to Paul that gun rights activists were concerned about their Constitutional rights, he was concerned about inner-city crime, a mass shooting in an elementary school and the right-wing nuts' unwillingness to recognize it was short-sighted and manipulated by the NRA.

And as Paul looked out the window, beyond his church and to the horizon, he asked himself, *Could I be wrong? Are they right? What makes me the final arbiter?*

Before the news returned to the screen, Paul asked his youngest child her opinion. "What makes us so right and others so wrong?"

Alyson looked from the screen to her Dad, stopped dictating imaginary letters to parents of children and constructing her Dad's eulogy and answered her Dad's question with a question. "I don't understand the question. Are you suggesting I think I'm always the smartest person in the room?"

"No. I'm not suggesting you're anything but open-minded. I just wonder how much any of us are willing to listen. I was raised by liberal parents who believed Franklin Roosevelt was without fault and used the government to protect people and promote fairness. They were peaceful and had no tolerance for violence. Because they were liberal and peaceful, I am liberal and peaceful as are you, your brother and sister."

Alyson was confused, but believed the answer would be presented if she was patient. She was inclined to interrupt, to ask *What?*, to pace, explore and peel the layers of the riddle, but she waited for her dying father to explain.

"And we're Christian. We believe we'll be rewarded in the here-after, because we believe that Jesus died for our sins. Why do we believe that? Not because Jesus told us to believe, not because he's sent clues for us to follow to his Cross, but because we were born and raised in Anoka, Minnesota. Everyone in Anoka is Christian. Not because they have been enlightened with evidence, but because their parents were Christian, their neighbors are Christian and when you turn on the television or radio and listen to a religious broadcast, it's a Christian broadcast. How many Christians live in Iraq? Very few. Not because Mohammed spoke to them or sent a written invitation, but because they were raised by Muslims, because they live in cities filled with Muslims and their neighborhoods are dotted with Mosques."

After Paul spoke, the philosophical question he asked was clearer and more interesting to Alyson. She signed her name to the imaginary letters she had composed to parents and folded the imaginary eulogy she had written into thirds and put it in her pretend pocket. With distractions neutralized, she listened more closely to what her dying father said.

"The truth is relative and is influenced by environment. Jesus is real to me, but not to Amir, who was born in Pakistan. Gun control is appropriate from my perspective, but to an impoverished black kid in Chicago, it's irrelevant and wrong, if it means he can't buy a gun on the street to protect his vulnerable Mom and younger siblings. I believe the government should be active and intervene to help the less fortunate, but tell that to an orphan who lost his parents while they waited for medical care and were unable to obtain it, because doctors in their community treated only those with private insurance and not those who presented Medicare Cards."

Alyson understood and smiled.

"Trump. No question, he's an egocentric clown, but to bright, neglected, quiet, people without hope and personal histories without mainstream answers, he's a possibility."

"I think you're going too far now."

"No. I'm not. They believe in Mohammed. They believe in unfettered access to guns, small government and Donald Trump. I disagree, but who am I to say, I'm right and they're wrong? Because I was born to liberal parents in a town where everyone was either Catholic or Lutheran? It's all relative. We're all right. It depends on our perspective."

"So, are you saying truth is relative?"

"It can be. If any interpretation is required, the truth is relative. Some facts are subject to interpretation. Some facts require no interpretation. The temperature is the temperature. If it's 30 degrees it 30 degrees. Doesn't matter who you are, it's 30 degrees. Where the air sits on the thermometer is not relative, it is what it is. But, whether it's cold or not, is subject to interpretation, and as a result, the truth about cold is relative. In the winter after a stretch of 25 below, when temperatures reach 20 above, it's not cold, it's unseasonably warm. At least to those of us who shivered through the deep freeze. But tell a guy from the Congo, sitting on the Equator that 20 above isn't cold, and he'll tell you, you're a liar. And from his perspective, he's right."

"And you just figured this out, on your death-bed?"

"No. I think I've always known it. It's just coming into better focus now. Studying the Bible as a kid, was an academic exercise. We read, we memorized and were tested. Jesus was just another quadratic equation. Now, it counts. Soon, I may be able to apply the lessons learned in Sunday School. Thousands of times I read and recited, *No one comes to the Father except through me?* And I've confessed my faith. Is it enough? If so, what about that guy who was raised in Islamabad, who was never given an opportunity to read the Bible or confess his Christian faith. His truth is different than mine. And it's not that I'm right and he's wrong. It isn't that simple. That truth is relative. I go to Heaven because I was raised in Anoka and he goes to Hell because he was raised in Islamabad? Nonsensical."

Alyson stood, resting her hands on the hospital bed side-rails. She furrowed her brow remembering what she was taught on

Sunday after Sunday after Sunday. "Are you saying we wasted our time on Sunday mornings?"

"No. The lessons you learned, the lessons I learned, are important, certainly here on earth, and maybe in the hereafter. Sunday School helped teach you the difference between right and wrong. It helped mold you into the good and caring woman you are. And maybe, what you learned will benefit you after you draw your last breath. I just don't know. And I'm too close to the answer to reject all those things I was taught to believe. I'm dying; I'm not stupid. The drugs have numbed the pain, not the fear factor. I'm not going to reject what I've been taught in Sunday School and church services minutes before the pay-off. No sense in doing that."

"You never were a gambler." Alyson fanned an imaginary poker hand, smiled at the cards she saw, closed the five pretend cards to a small stack and tossed them to the non-existent card-table. "Fold."

"I don't think it's gambling. There's no pay-off in rejecting Christianity at this stage. At 15, huge pay-off, at 25, big pay-off, at 45, significant pay-off, at 65, pay-off, now, in bed, dying, no pay-off. I can no longer enjoy the fruits of sin. Can't steal another man's riches or enjoy his wife. It's too late for me. And in case He's listening, I'm not rejecting Christianity. Everything I was taught, everything you were taught, every verse from the Bible we read and memorized, may be truth. I'm not denying it, I'm simply suggesting that it's arrogant and insensitive to disparage a Muslim for not understanding Christianity. And I don't think God would either."

"So, then, what is religious truth?"

"I don't know. I'm not that smart. Maybe none of it; maybe all of it. But, that's not my point. My point is, truth can be relative. When we say Jesus is the only answer and all others who claim to be the *Answer* are false profits, I'm telling Muslims, that they're wrong and Jews that they're wrong, and I'm not so sure. I'm not only not sure, I understand why they disagree, and accept that their truth is different than mine and that it may be in every respect as valid as mine."

"And Trump?"

"That's a little more difficult. I can accept that Muslim and Jews may be right, that Christians may be wrong, but it's more difficult to conclude those who support Trump are right on any level." Paul laughed. He felt strongly about Trump, but didn't equate him with Satan or anti-Christianity. The distaste was powerful, but not overwhelming. Paul's laugh morphed into a cough and then, the need to expel expectorant. After spitting chunks in a napkin and dropping it into the waste basket attached to the side of his bed, Paul completed his thought.

"It's difficult, but I think I get it. I think he's a childish, idiotic, egocentric jerk; they see him as an alternative, an alternative that is absolutely necessary to change direction, to avoid catastrophe. For them, his ego and egocentricity are irrelevant, or at least, unimportant. Like you, like me, they want what's best and happen to believe he can deliver it. They think we're in danger. Bush, Obama, Clinton, all the same. They can't afford to feed their families, can't find rewarding work, can't pay the medical bills or obtain affordable medical insurance, can't pay the rent or mortgage, can't retire, even at age 75, can't compete with African-Americans who are fed with food stamps, are housed in federally subsidized housing and were educated at impressive colleges where their tuition was paid by a government grant designed to close the gap between White and Black, a gap whose existence they refuse to accept. All of Trump's predecessors have promised them the same thing, prosperity and security, but have failed to deliver. And now, those same politicians, are ignoring them, speaking instead to Mexicans, Muslims, those with newly accepted sexual preferences, professional women and those who are young, bright, untarnished by failure and look forward to a prosperous future. Trump says, *Screw all of those clowns, follow me.* And he's different. Inarticulate. Apolitical. Coarse. Entertaining."

Paul paused to gather wind. He'd not said so many words at once in a while. It was tiring, but he needed to finish. It was important, a commitment to open-mindedness, a pledge to understanding others. "His message and his manner convince the disaffected that he's different, their guy. I get it. Based on what they've experienced, based on their hopes, he's the answer. Not mine, but theirs. And for them, it's true. Some truths are relative. And for them, Trump is truly the best answer."

Maybe near-death provided Paul with the ability to disassociate and see things as he couldn't when he was worried about his mortgage, his children, his health, his future. Self-preservation was moot. But now, he was a brain in a jar. It didn't matter to him if it rained, snowed, hailed, dipped below zero or soared beyond 100. If the sun failed to rise, *So what?* If clocks stopped and work days stretched to 12 hours, *Who cares?* A fire in California? A flood in Japan? Earthquakes? Economic collapse, records highs for the DOW, terrorist attacks in Paris? *Okay, why do I care?* He wasn't as invested in the world as he was poised to leave it. Maybe it helped him see things from another perspective.

When Trump asked to see President Obama's birth certificate, Alyson told Paul, she was suspicious of his intent. When he announced he would run, she was suspicious of his intentions, saying, *He doesn't want to win, he wants the publicity* and scoffed at his chances saying, *He can't win, no one will take him seriously*. After listening to the rational rant of a dying man, unchained from selfishness by death's presence, she wondered. "Can he win?"

"No. Not a chance. He's crazy. The window to his world is a mirror. He's a nut. He can't win. But, at least we understand why his supporters support him. And because some truths may relative, they may be right."

chapter ten

I n spite of his best efforts to remain engaged, after a taxing conversation which required heavy lifting, Paul drifted to sleep. As a young man, he spent hours in the courtroom sparring with opponents and judges, seemingly finding nuggets of clarity in statutes, rules and decisions written in legalize and misunderstood since publication, and after the day in court, met with clients and witnesses and prepared for the next day's battle. After 14 hour work days, he walked into the house with a smile and bounce in his step, kissed Mary, hugged the kids, helped with homework, often explaining complicated math he didn't understand when a math student, watched the news, read part of a book and fell asleep still sharp, still wide awake. He was young then. Not so now. After twenty minutes of television news and a conversation it spawned, a conversation about Trump, religion and open-mindedness, Paul was exhausted and unable to fight the urge to sleep. He slept.

When he opened his eyes, it was still light. *Today? Tomorrow?* It didn't matter, he was still there. Belle sat on the chair next to his bed. "Hello."

Paul combed his hair with his fingers. He was emaciated, gray, old and dying, yet he combed his hair with his fingers. *Habit? Vanity? Vanity.* "How long was I out?"

Belle stood and moved a stubborn strand of hair from Paul's forehead to the top of his head, where it wrestled with the more compliant locks. "Not long. About an hour."

Paul pushed the bed-button and as the head of his bed rose, the non-conformist gray hair that had ignored the dictates of a hand that served as a comb, aided by gravity, fell to his forehead. Tickled by the strand that was unwilling to lie down with others, Paul plucked the celibate from his scalp, scratched his forehead and smiled. "Good. I don't want to sleep it away."

Belle smiled. "Anything I can get you?"

"Nope."

As Belle turned to leave Paul's cell, his oasis, Paul cleared his old and failing throat and to the extend he could, called out to the hall and those who waited for their opportunity to reminisce with a dying man. "Next."

Paul was glad he and Mary reconfigured their home when they aged. They installed a ramp and widened the doorways so Mary could come and go comfortably, after she replaced a hip and fell and broke a leg while recovering. Paul looked to the wide doorway and watched Pinky Little's 55-year-old daughter wheel Pinky into the room. After she pushed Pinky's wheelchair to the side of Paul's bed and rotated it so Pinky faced Paul, she said, "I'll be in the living room with Mary and the others, let me know when you want to leave." As the unmarried, squatty woman walked from the room, Paul confirmed the need for wide doorways.

Paul surveyed his old friend. A leather strap tied him to the chair in which he sat. The chest belt kept him upright. His head leaned forward, pulling his neck, shoulders and chest towards his knees. Without the leather strap, Pinky would have fallen forward, out of the chair and onto the carpet. His mouth was agape, his eyes swollen and red and his hands shaking and blue. He wore a catheter, a waste bag and scars on his arms, mapping the veins into which medicine had been injected for decades.

Pinky was a survivor, a fighter, an anomaly. He was diagnosed with cancer at 40, had a stroke at 52, two heart attacks by 64, Crones disease, bypass surgery twice, Parkinson's, cancer at 68 and a calcium deficiency that resulted in broken bones when he fell, banged a toe or stood too quickly. His doctors gave him six months to live at 40, a year at 65, 30 days at 68 and now, they just smiled.

Paul was scheduled to die in days, and yet, he was the healthiest man in the room. He wasn't certain if Pinky had come to comfort him or had come for comfort. "How are you, Pinky?"

Pinky slowly lifted his limping head from his chest, looked at Paul and smiled. "Good. I feel good. You?"

Paul marveled at his resolve, his fight, his optimism. In spite of a body that resisted smooth skin, a straight back, digestion, a strong, steady heartbeat and willingly invited cancer, viruses and decay, he smiled, appreciated what he had today and looked forward to what he'd have tomorrow. It wouldn't be much, but it'd be enough for Pinky. He had come to comfort, not be comforted. Paul answered Pinky's question and challenge. "You know how it is. Dying and old. But, frankly, I feel pretty good too. Can't eat, constantly tired, lungs hurt, hard to breathe, chained to my bed or chair on wheels, but I feel pretty good."

As Pinky listened to Paul's answer, his head slowly descended to his chest, and when Paul stopped talking, signaling the need for a response from Pinky, his head bobbed to the surface and he mumbled. Paul had listened to Pinky's mumbling for decades, since childhood. He had experience. Paul didn't need for Pinky to enunciate or speak more loudly; he understood. "Don't listen to the doctors. They don't know what they're talking about. If I'd ov listened, I'd been dead for 35-years. And look, here I am. Ready for the race."

"What race is that, Pinky?"

"Oh, I don't know. The space race? Race relations? The rat race? I don't know; I'm just here, still breathing, still contributing."

"When the doctors told you, you were going to die, did you ever believe it?"

Paul's question was short; it hadn't given Pinky's head enough time to descend to his chest. Once the downward motion began, it was destined to complete its journey, so Pinky answered while his head dropped and rebounded, modulating the loudness of his answer. "Nope. Never. They said, *You're going to die,* and

I said, *Screw you*. Never believed them. I told them they were wrong. They smiled, loved my pluck, but smiled that arrogant, I'm-smarter-than-you-smile and left, believing they'd see me buried around the block. Well guess what? I'm still here, and those doctors who predicted my death, they're dead. Poetry."

Pinky was a custodian. He never left high school. He was a student on June fifth, and on the sixth, he was given keys to the building and taught how to monitor the boiler, operate a floor-buffer, push a broom, clean toilets and empty waste baskets. He earned a livable wage, took two-weeks of vacation a year, contributed to a pension and liked his work. As he worked with an ear bud connected to a transistor radio, he listened to the Twins in the spring, summer and fall and the Gophers and fifties music in the winters. His life was unrewarding, yet simple, secure and sweet.

Paul and Pinky were raised in the same neighborhood. They attended the same elementary school, junior high and high school and graduated the same year. When Paul obtained his driver's license and purchased a car, he picked Pinky up and drove him to and from school. They were friends who learned to smoke together and shared alcohol stolen from their fathers. When 13, when things began to stir in their pants, they shared magazines and fantasies.

Five years after he began working for the School District, Pinky called his friend, who was a first-year law student and sought his counsel. "Paul, I've got an opportunity to buy a business. I'm not sure what I should do."

"What kind of business?"

"A restaurant. Fast food. It's part of a chain."

"You don't know anything about owning a restaurant."

"I know, but they say they'll teach me."

"Who?"

"The company guys. They say they've done it before and will be happy to do it again."

"Why you?"

"My sister, who lives in California suggested it, I told her I was interested and next thing I know, they called."

"How much money?"

"Well, that's the interesting part. A guy I know wants to invest. He thinks this company has a good future. He wants to be my silent partner. He'll put up the money, I'll pay him back with interest and a percentage of the profits and if things go according to the plan, he'll be paid off in ten years and he'll bow out. It seems like a good idea. What do you think?"

Paul held the phone to his ear, closed his eyes and pictured Pinky in the high school hallways, with a transistor radio connected to his ear by a white chord, a broom in his hand and a smile on his face. He visualized a life without anxiety, a life with early retirement and vacations in the sun and compared that life with one fraught with unknowns, corporate in-fighting, long hours, employee issues and failed investments, and answered the question his friend had asked. "Stay at the school. Too many unknowns. You've got it pretty good now."

Pinky ignored his friend's advice and purchased a McDonald's franchise. When the doctors told him, he had cancer at 40, Pinky owned eight restaurants, and when he sold his business interests after his second heart attack, he owned 17 stores and banked over twenty-million dollars. Paul represented Pinky in the transaction, and when the closer handed Pinky a certified check, he looked at Paul and said, *Stay at the school?*

"Pinky, you ever regret leaving the school and buying restaurants?"

"Not really. I made a lot of money with McDonalds. Sometimes, I wonder if the work made me sick. There was a lot of pressure. Lots of money, lots of deals, lots of pressure. I was always on edge, always looking for the next location, always leveraging my position, always fighting off competition, always looking over my shoulder. I hired managers and they did good work, but it was always my name, my money, my decision. And with lots of stores and lots of employees, there were lots of crises. It took a toll."

Pinky let his head fall and bob up twice, as if his head was a pump handle that needed to go up and down and up, to extract energy and words from a well below. Replenished, he finished his analysis. "The money was great. My family and the families they create, all down the line, won't need to worry about money; I made enough for all of them, but, pushing a broom while listening to Harmon Killebrew hit and Camilo Pasqual pitch or Bobby Darin sing, was pretty good. The broom didn't fight back and the school district never asked me decide if a manager was sexually inappropriate to another employee. It was easy, uneventful, peaceful. I made money, but at what cost? Look at me. Look at us. Maybe if I'd have stayed with my broom and you'd have joined me in the boiler room, we'd be on the golf course now and not in a hospice bed or wheelchair. Maybe you were right when you suggested I stay at the school. Who knows? But nothing can be done now my friend."

Paul coughed and then Pinky coughed. "Catchy, like yawning."

"No Paul, we're old and dying. I didn't follow suit, I didn't cough because you did; I did what my old lungs and scratchy throat required me to do."

The men were silent, Paul confined to his bed by sickness and side rails and Pinky confined to his chair by sickness and a leather strap. Paul thought about asking Pinky about his three kids, the one who tended to Pinky, the broad, old virgin who wheeled him to Paul, another, a man who attended pride rallies in South Minneapolis and lived with a man in an apartment with one bedroom and a third who gave Pinky three grandchildren, one of whom had purchased a Burger Chef franchise and often asked Grandpa for advice and money, but Paul knew Pinky's answer would be, *All fine, all healthy, all where they should be and with the ones they love*, so he didn't ask.

As the silence lingered, it became uncomfortable. There were no more pretenses between the old friends, pretenses had died years before cancer visited Pinky, but the men understood time was short, that others wanted to share memories with a dying man and that their silence deprived them both of meaningful intercourse. As Pinky was about to tell his old friend *Goodbye* for the last time, a flicker ignited something in a box of memories closed for years. His head remained upright, his eyes cleared, the corners of his mouth pitched towards his ears and he looked at his fellow traveler. "Do you remember Mr. Dalbec?"

"The English teacher?"

"Yeah."

Paul remembered. He was young. He taught 10th grade English when Paul and Pinky were tenth graders and left for California at the end of the school year. "I remember his goodbye. On the last day of school, he told our class, it had been a pleasure to have taught us, but that he was suffocating in a small town in Minnesota. As I recall, he told us that when the school bell sounded, he'd get in his car and drive west until he could drive no more. He said, *If my paycheck finds me, so be it and if not, so be that as well.* And when the bell rang, we watched him walk to the parking lot, climb behind the wheel of his packed Bel Air and drive away. Never heard of or from him again. Why'd you bring him up."

Pinky smiled. He was 34, breathing salt air and listening to waves lap the shore. His wheelchair had disappeared, his lungs were clear, his bones strong and cancer, was something that had happened to others, not him. "I saw him in California. 1968. Ray Kroc had a shindig for franchise owners in San Diego. The night after Bobby Kennedy was killed, I was drinking in a hotel bar, thinking that nothing mattered anymore. JFK, Martin Luther King and then Bobby. I was depressed. Ray Kroc had tried to rally the troops, but how could I be enthusiastic about hamburgers when bullets were robbing us of our future?"

"All of those guys, dead for more than 40 years, weren't much older than us, Pink."

"I know. A terrible shame. So, I'm in this bar, getting drunk, and I look at the bartender and think he looks familiar. Do you know who it was?"

"Well, because I've already been told the subject of this story, I can fathom a guess."

"Mr. Dalbec."

"Really?"

"Yeah, really."

Paul was impressed by Pinky's memory and the strength it brought to his neck. His head remained atop a neck that was perpendicular to the floor. No dipping, no bobbing. Upright. Still.

"So, I look at him and say, *Mr. Dalbec.* Do you know what he said?"

"Pinky?"

"No. He wasn't my teacher. He didn't know who I was. He said, *I am and you're from Minnesota.* I was drunk, so easy to impress, but I was impressed that he didn't know me but could divine that I was from Minnesota. When I asked how he knew I was from Minnesota, he said, *Because your skin is pale, like you've been indoors and out of the sun and cold for months, and no one calls me Mr. Dalbec and never has, except students I taught in Minnesota. Am I right?* He was and I told him so."

"A bartender?"

"Yeah. He said he was trying to find himself and that bartending gave him an opportunity to meet different people in a relaxed setting. He told me he hated the cold and structure that compromised him in Minnesota. He seemed really happy. Because the bar was kinda empty, he stood in front of me while I sat at the bar and drank. When the bar closed, he asked if I wanted to get something to eat and we went to a 24-hour café that shared a parking lot with a McDonald's owned by Kroc. After we ate, I went with him to his place and met his roommate. Good guy. And then he told me he was homosexual. He said he was gay, but in 68, I had no idea what that meant. Happy? I didn't know. When he saw that I didn't get it, he made it clear. *Homosexual*."

Paul was unimpressed. In 2015, heterosexual mayors marched with their wives in *Gay Pride* parades, men married men with the blessing of the courts and lesbians were able to succeed in court if they convinced a jury that they were treated differently, because of their sexual orientation. In 1968, homosexuals hid their orientation, but Paul was smart enough to know, they were always there, waiting to be heard. "Doesn't shock me. When you say it, thinking back, it fits. Not surprising."

Pinky tried to lift his butt from his chair, to straighten his back, but his arms were too weak, so he continued his story from a slouch. "Here's the interesting part of the story. I slept with Mr. Dalbec and his roommate that night. And I don't mean, fell asleep. We kissed, moaned, did all the things gay men do with one another. Twice. He took me to the airport the next afternoon, on his way to the bar. I was tempted to ask him if I could stay a couple more days, but didn't. I got on the plane and never heard from him again."

Paul pushed the bed-button and sat straight up. Shocked, caught off-guard, looking at a man he had looked at for nearly 70-years and seeing someone different, Paul could only muster, "Huh?"

"It was the only time ever. And I've never told anyone, ever. You are the only one. I figure, you're safe. You don't have access to a computer or telephone and I'm guessing you don't want to spend your last few days outing an old man in a wheelchair."

Paul coughed, reached for a tissue in which he spat a piece of his lung, remembered where he was and why, and regained his composure. "I didn't think anyone could make me forget that I'm dying. You did that my friend. Touché."

"There were days I wondered, days I remembered what I did in San Diego, but never acted on my memories. I was married, had three kids and a wonderful wife. Things were great in our bedroom. I blamed it on Bobby Kennedy's assassination, booze and Mr. Dalbec. But, when I thought about it, I never felt shame, never guilt. And when I let my memories get graphic, I was always a little aroused. Not flat out hard, but a little stiff. Maybe in a different time, a different generation, things would have been different. But it wasn't a different time, so it was one night. No more, no less. Surprised? Offended?"

"I'm too old and too close to the other side to judge, Pinky. Earlier today, I told Aly that truth can be relative. Your story is a perfect example. In 1963, a man kissing a man was wrong, sick, shameful. Those kinds of desires were to be denied and if they persisted, a priest, pastor or psychologist was called and asked to exorcise the desires or strengthen the commitment to deny them. And now, men marry men, women marry women and therapists who *treat homosexuality* are considered borderline crazy. The truth about homosexuality has morphed. The truth has changed. I won't judge, except to the extent you're looking for exoneration, absolution. I doubt you need my approval, but if you do, you have it. I don't care what happened in 1968 or what you've considered since then. You're a good man and have always been a good man."

"Maybe I was looking for approval. I don't know. I don't know why I told you. After 37 years? I don't know. Maybe maintaining silence was a burden. Keep quiet, deny the truth and hide from what you did, who you are. And now I've told someone. It was a pretty eventful evening and hiding it from everyone was denying something important. No more. The cuffs are off. You know and I'm liberated."

Paul smiled at his old crippled friend. He was unable to leave his chair, unable to use a toilet, unable to show affection for a woman or a man. "Memories are what we have my friend. If the memory makes you happy, share it, embrace it."

Pinky's energy was depleted by recalling the encounter that excited him then, and aroused him mildly thereafter, and his head dipped to his chest. Paul couldn't see his mouth, but knew he was smiling, freed at last. Pinky coughed, swallowed expectorant and wiped his wet smiling mouth with the sleeve of his faded shirt. "So, now you know."

Paul reached for his friend's hand which rested on a rubber wheel, but his arms were too short, his reach insufficient. "Do you know what happened to Mr. Dalbec?"

Answering his friend, but speaking to his chest, Pinky said, "No. Recently, just curious, I tried to look him up on the internet, but without a first name, it provided no clues. Lots of Dalbecs in San Diego."

Paul whispered. "Your man lover, and you don't know his first name?"

"Nope. It didn't matter then and it doesn't now. Didn't know then, don't know now. In my dreams, if I had them, and I make no admission, I moaned, *Mr. Dalbec*. And for what it's worth, I don't think he ever knew my first or last name. Just a kid, now a young man, from Anoka. Names were unimportant, irrelevant."

After more comfortable silence, Pinky lifted his chin from his chest, muffled a cough, smiled and offered his confidant a small, shaking hand. When the two old hands forged a precarious, vulnerable bridge between the dying lawyer and the businessman who continued to cheat death, a bridge between 1968 and 2015, between truth as it was and truth as it existed then, Pinky cleared his throat, opened his mouth to gather enough air to speak and said, "Goodbye, my friend. See you on the other side."

chapter eleven

Paul was tired, yet awake and unable to sleep. Electrified by discovery, surprised by his old friend's admission, he couldn't sleep. When he closed his eyes, he pictured Pinky holding hands with a man, kissing him and moaning, and was startled to consciousness. He wasn't repulsed, wasn't in the least bit offended by Pinky's night of infidelity, just surprised. *You think you know someone, know them for 70 years and discover, you don't know something significant, defining. Surprising. Shocking. Wow.*

Belle returned to the room, asked Paul if he needed anything and when Paul told her, *the next person in line*, she disappeared and Mary appeared in her place.

"How was Pinky?"

"He was Pinky. I'm not sure who's sicker, him or me."

Mary stood near Paul, bent over the bed, so her face was close to Paul's and whispered. "Paula says the doctors told him, his time is short. Told him not to venture from home, that unnecessary movement and activity will hasten his death."

"Paula's too dramatic, maybe looking for her inheritance. He seemed pretty good to me. And even if the doctors told him what she said, they've been telling him that for 35 years. He's defied the odds and outlived their predictions for a long time. I'd put my money on him, not the doctors."

"He looked pretty sick, but he always does. When he left, he had a big grin on his face. What'd you talk about?"

"Just old man talk. He probably was smiling, because he figured he was in good shape, relatively speaking. He's old, been condemned early and often, but today, he spent time with an old friend whose life expectancy is shorter than his. Probably made him feel a little better. But, to be honest, when I saw him, strapped to that chair, with his head bobbing up and down and his frail hands shaking, I felt pretty good about where I am in life. It's all relative."

Mary adjusted Paul's pillow so that his head rested on its middle, covered his left hand with both of hers and asked, "Ready for more? The kitchen is full."

"Who's here?"

"All of the kids. I think they're here for the duration, which I hope is months long. And Sandy James, Tom Pertler and Rex Boyd."

Rex was their next-door neighbor, who was 86 and looked and acted like he was 65. When Paul was first diagnosed, Rex asked his grandson to plow Paul's driveway, and when spring appeared, he started his lawn mower, and when he reached the west end of his lot, the place where he typically turned and created the next strip of cut grass, he kept right on going, until he reached the west end of Paul's lot. When Rex had finished mowing his yard, he had finished mowing Paul's. He didn't ask, didn't explain, he just did. Three times a week, Rex knocked on the door and when Mary answered, he asked, *Anything you need?*

A widower, Paul thought Rex was interested in Mary. Even when he talked about the grass, the snow or cluttered gutters, subjects about which men talk, he directed his words to Mary. When Mary smiled, Rex smiled. When Mary laughed, Rex laughed. If Mary asked a question, Rex listened, heard and responded promptly and with a smile. If Paul asked a question, Rex asked one as well, *I'm sorry, what did you say Paul?*

Since he was committed to his bedroom, Paul thought he heard Rex's voice and laughter in the kitchen often. Rarely did Rex look in on Paul; he laughed and talked in the kitchen with Mary. Paul surprised himself when his ears began to burn and attributed the aberrant blood flow to jealousy. He was on his back, unable to stand, unable to hug his wife, unable to defend himself or the sanctity of their marriage, unable to confront his rival with clenched fists or aggressive language. Rex was an 86 year old widower, with titanium hips, a pacemaker, failing vision which made it impossible for him to appreciate Mary's elegant, mature beauty, and likely, erectile dysfunction, and yet Paul was jealous.

"Rex isn't here to see me. He's here for you. And even if he was here to see me, he's at the bottom of my list."

Sandy James was a young associate pastor at Zion Lutheran. The Church sent Drake Milford to the house when Paul first received the news that he was dying. Drake was the Senior Pastor of the church with 2,500 baptized members. He was busy overseeing his flock and managing his large staff. When days stretched into weeks and weeks into months, when the inevitable was clearly not imminent, Drake stopped visiting and Sandy appeared. She was pleasant and clearly driven by the forces that directed her to the Seminary, service and compassion, but Paul wanted to spend time with Sandy, when it was time. He wanted her close, in the event fear nibbled at his convictions and compromised his confidence. It wasn't that time.

"Send in Tom."

Tom Pertler was a disbarred lawyer. He clerked for Paul when he was a law student and worked for a small firm in Anoka after he passed the bar. He was kind, generous, disorganized. He tried, but couldn't overcome his inability to organize. His calendar was incomplete, and incomprehensible, his files, a mess and his ability to fix mess and confusion, non-existent. He was always late for court and oftentimes, didn't make appearances, because he didn't remember he was supposed to be in court or when. He hired legal assistants who tried to manage his calendar and get him to court on time, but because they were not in the courtroom when hearings were scheduled, they needed to rely on Tom for information to make their management effective. They couldn't; Tom was unreliable.

Maybe it was his father, who showed little, if any affection. Maybe it was a missing chromosome that helped organize the lives of others and in its absence, not Tom. Maybe it was poor upbringing or a traumatic event. Whatever it was, it was. In spite of his best efforts, Tom couldn't do it as required.

When the demands of clients and the courts became overwhelming, when it was clear that a failure to do as required would jeopardize Tom's ability to practice law in the future, he began to lie. Tom looked, concluded dishonesty was his only option and fibbed in an attempt to survive. He told courts he was late because he was ill or his mother had died, told clients the Court had rescheduled without telling him, and other lawyers, that court administration had suggested no hearing was necessary. When he told a Judge in Hennepin County that he hadn't appeared because his mother was gravely ill and that Judge recalled that a year earlier, Tom had explained an unexcused absence with his mother's unexpected death, the fraud was discovered and Tom was done.

The Lawyers Board investigated Tom. His trust account was illegible and money was missing, without explanation. His files were disorganized and replete with unfiled documents that were tardy and incomplete. When the investigators called Tom's clients, they all vouched for his kindness and good intentions, but expressed frustration with his communications, efforts and accounting.

When the investigation was complete, the Board found 22 violations and recommended disbarment. Tom wasn't interested in contesting the allegations, recognizing most were true, and knew he would never overcome his deficiencies, his inability to appropriately organize, to keep good records and manage money that wasn't his, would never be able to practice law again without being haunted by his unseemly history, so agreed to disbarment. Quick. Easy. When he received a copy of the Supreme Court's Order, the one that stripped him of his ability to practice law, Tom smiled. He was accused and convicted, yet rescued and freed. He exhaled the tension and anxiety and smiled.

Without a license to practice law, Tom looked for work in areas unrelated to the law, but every time he disclosed that he was a disbarred lawyer, prospective employers, smiled, shook his hand, told him they'd give him a call later and didn't. He moved into his mother's home at 38, and after she called her late husband's best friend, the local Postmaster, he began to haul mail.

Letter carriers need organization to survive the Post Office. Trays of unsorted mail, mounds of envelopes filled with letters, some big, some small, some addressed clearly and others, illegible, needed to be filed in assigned slots in each carrier's box, removed from the box, bound, stacked in a mail bag according to destination and ultimately deposited in mailboxes with numbers that corresponded to the numbers on the envelopes. It required organizational skills that Tom lacked naturally, but the Post Office tools and routine simplified the process and so long as Tom followed the rules, arrived at 6:00 a.m., and stifled conversation until his mail was sorted and packed, he was able to do as the Post Office wanted.

Paul's home was on Tom's postal route. If Paul was home when the mail arrived, Tom knocked, stopped and had coffee with Paul. If Paul wasn't home when Tom delivered letters, he attached a message scribbled on a post-it note, to a piece of junk mail, and there was always junk mail. The messages were like the mailman, sweet and kind. *Have a good day my friend. Enjoy. It's Saturday, enjoy the time off. It's Monday, don't let the work week get you down. Have a good day Paul. It's me, who else? Smile.* As a lawyer, he was tardy by nature and acerbic by design, a late arriving contentious advocate. As a mailman, he was kind, sharing a smile and upbeat messages at every opportunity. The Post Office uniform fit better than the white shirt and tie.

They never discussed the law. They shared a distaste for litigation, *stare decisis*, cumbersome statutes, the absence of commonsense solutions, people arguing about things too small to be worthy of argument, judges who dispensed justice with a heavy hand and empty mind, discourteous, aggressive opposing counsel and courtroom pretenses. Tom left it behind when the Lawyers Board told him he had no choice and Paul escaped after 40-years, when he retired. Both left what they didn't like and had no interest in returning.

Tom walked into Paul's hospice, his cell, wearing his summer uniform. His face was tan, his legs and arms bare and his smile broad. When he practiced law, he was tight, his mouth pursed and his brow ever furrowed. As he said *Hello* to his former mentor, the marks of anxiety had been erased and existed only in memory. He was relaxed, happy and bounced as he walked.

"Did you bring my mail?"

"I did. I left it with Mary. Renewal notice from the Bar Association. Better pay it soon or you'll owe a penalty."

"I'll tell Mary right away. Can't die with an expired membership. How are you?"

Tom framed himself with his hands and pointed to his face which sported an exaggerated, wide grin. "I'm great. I get paid to walk six miles a day and bring people Christmas Cards, birthday cards, presents, great deals described in circulars and an occasional bill. I'm Santa without the sleigh. It's a wonderful life. I'm good. How about you?"

"Still here. Given the circumstances, I can't complain. I visit with people, sleep, dream of my past and dread the end, but, I'm at peace with it. As Doris Day said, *Que sera sera*. Too late to change the outcome now."

"If you can't change the outcome, why do priests show up for last rites?"

"You'd need to ask a Catholic. Me, I'm a wayward Lutheran. Our religious leader drops by to provide comfort, not salvation. I think she believes salvation has already been assured. God, I hope so."

"You and I, we've already been to Hell. It was a courtroom, in Stearns County. No need to return. We've done our time. Salvation assured."

Tom laughed, but the best Paul could do, was muster a smile. Paul appreciated his friend's willingness to laugh at death, but its nearness made it difficult for him to laugh. Tom was young, likely 30 years from Paul's bed. It was easy for him to laugh about the death riddle, he wouldn't be required to formulate an answer for three decades. When Paul was Tom's age, when his health was as Tom's was on the day he smiled at his friend who laid in a bed with side-rails, he joked about passing. *I'll tell St. Peter, the check's in the mail.* It was funny, death was remote, a consequence to be experienced years away. *I can atone, make changes, do good things, save my soul. There's plenty of time. No hurry.* That time had passed. No chance to atone; no chance to do good things and save his soul. *Que sera, sera.*

"I guess I'll know soon enough."

"Well, my friend, I'm confident that the discovery will be a good one. If anyone deserves a pleasant passage and eternal happiness, it's you."

"I'm not quite that confident. If I had a playbook, I'd study it hard and do what I could to please my teachers."

"Isn't that the Bible?"

"It's a book. I'm not sure it's the playbook. They have a different one across the ocean and yet another, in Utah. I don't know. I have my suspicions, but I'm not certain."

"As you know, I've never been much good at organizing my thoughts and making decisions. If you're looking for answers, ask someone who was able to keep their license to practice law, not me. I'm clueless."

"No, you're not. You are one of the few who had the courage to reject what didn't fit. You didn't lose your license, you gave it away. And that was a good thing."

Tom didn't need to hear it from Paul. He knew it. He confirmed the wisdom of his choice every night when he fell asleep fast, without regret, without fear, without dread. He confirmed the wisdom of his sacrifice every morning when he woke from deep, restful sleep with a smile and when he whistled while he showered. His decision to leave law and forfeit his license was the best decision he had made. He knew it. "Thank you, my friend. Get your rest. Others are here to see you. I'll make way and see you tomorrow. Same time, same place."

Tom touched Paul's left arm, attached a post-it note to the bedside table that read, *Smile, it's worth the effort*, and walked from the room, leaving Paul alone with his thoughts. His eyes closed and he drifted to a place other than his bedroom. A large, black man wearing a clerical collar, Yamaka and carrying a Torah, spoke from behind a Buddhist statue. *Riches. Best not measure riches by the square footage of your home, the depth of your bank accounts or the origin of the leather in your shoes. Those things are unimportant and unworthy of the chase. Riches. It's peace of mind, smiles and comfortable shoes.*

Mary walked into the bedroom with Sandy James, who wore a clerical collar and a concerned look. She wondered if the motionless, old, wrinkled, shrinking man in the bed, under the covers, had died. As the two women shared panic looks, like a man suffering from apnea, Paul gasped air with a snort and began to breath comfortably. Mary relaxed, smiled, looked at Pastor James and said, "Maybe tomorrow."

Pastor James was startled, surprised by Mary's cavalier reference to Paul's impending end. "Maybe he'll die tomorrow?"

Mary smiled and disarmed the modestly offended cleric. "No. Maybe tomorrow he'll be awake so that you can speak to him."

When the Pastor left the room, Mary sat on the bedside chair and read *A Prayer for Owen Meany*. As she turned pages, she looked at her husband and confirmed he was still breathing. After ten pages, she concluded everything was fine, as good as it could be, and left the bedroom.

Paul dreamed. He was on a beach surrounded by thousands, millions, maybe billions of dogs of all sizes and breeds. Cockers, Labs, Setters, Poodles, Dachshunds, Greyhounds, Retrievers, Basset Hounds and Beagles as far as he could see. They rolled in the sand, barked and moved to the music that was broadcast from the sun. It was a Beatles song, but Paul was unable to determine if it was *Hey Jude, Something* or *Yesterday*. Dogs nibbled at Paul's feet and when he walked in the direction of the blue water, they protested his movement by biting, snarling and barking in aggressive tones. When he arrived at the water's edge, Paul stepped into the water and cooled his feet, hot with dog bites.

As a haze that smelled of cinnamon descended from above, Paul looked to the sky, lost his balance and began to fall. Afraid the fall would break his brittle bones and kill the baby dogs that surrounded him, Paul lifted his legs so that he would land on his ample bottom, believing his soft toosh would cushion his landing and save puppies. *Splash.* The dogs disappeared and Paul sunk deep into the ocean. The water was frigid; Paul was cold. When he fell to the uneven, rocky, shell-lined bottom of the sea, Paul squatted and pushed himself toward the sun as hard as he could, rocketing through layers of water and past fish of a thousand colors. When he reached the surface, Paul drew a sharp, quick, deep breath, thought he heard a familiar voice, a mature woman's voice, say, *Maybe tomorrow,* and walked to the shoreline where his Dad waited.

"Well?"

Paul didn't understand. Was he asking about the puppies, the ocean floor or the familiar voice? "Well what?"

His Dad drew in a breath, held it and released it as he spoke. "Did you open your eyes under the water?"

Paul remembered. His Dad drove him to the ocean and asked him to swim under the water and open his eyes. He laughed while he told him he'd see fish, coral and beautiful shells in the water. "I did. And I didn't see anything. The salt burned my eyes. I couldn't keep them open, it hurt too much."

Paul's Dad laughed more loudly than before. "No fish?"

"No."

"No coral?"

"No."

"Beautiful shells? You must've seen beautiful shells. Did you see shells?"

"I didn't see anything. The salt stung my eyes."

"Well, I owe you a dollar. You did it, and I said if you did, I'd give you a buck. Remind me later."

His Dad handed Paul a beach towel, a large one with a picture of coral, fish and shells, and Paul wiped the salt out of his eyes.

When he dropped the towel to his feet and opened his salt-free eyes, he was on a football field, standing on the sidelines, wearing a football uniform that was too big for his stunted body. His small head swam in the helmet that repeatedly tipped forward and blocked his vision. Paul unsnapped the chinstrap, pulled the helmet from his head and dropped it to his feet. He could see. He was at Goodrich field, Anoka's football stadium, off the field, near the 50-yard line. He looked to his right and then his left. His teammates stood with him, dwarfed him and ridiculed him. *Fumbler. Loser. Pip squeak.*

As he was about to ask the large man-child who stood to his right, what he had done to deserve criticism, Paul's Dad emerged from the stands and answered questions Paul was about to ask someone else. "How could you? Your Mom and I are in the stands and you do that? Unbelievable. Drop the ball on the one-yard line? Unbelievable. You're an embarrassment."

Not remembering his error, but accepting its consequences, Paul looked to the turf, kicked chalk, inspected his palms, hands that lost the ball and apologized. "I'm sorry, Dad. I didn't try to drop the ball."

Looking through eyes clouded with an excess of salt-water, Paul watched his Dad wipe a tear from his cheek and shake his head. His Dad mumbled. Paul wasn't sure what he said, but he got the gist of it. *Clown, loser, embarrassment.*

Paul looked into the stands, in search of his mother, her compassion and forgiveness, but saw none of what he looked for. The concrete perches were empty, save a pile of civilian clothes and a helmet that read *Thomas 32*. When the coach called for Paul to enter the game and carry the ball, in search of redemption, Paul looked for his helmet at his feet, couldn't find it and ran to the stands to retrieve the helmet with his name and number, but when plucked it from the spectator bench and turned to field, the field was gone, as were his teammates. Only his Dad remained and he was sobbing, rubbing his red eyes with the knuckles of clenched fists. He was wailing. *Why me? Why did the interstate kill my business and ruin my reputation?*

As Paul walked to his Dad, as he formulated a speech that explained kismet and acquitted his father of wrongdoing, the grass became tile, the evening sky, a false white ceiling with bright lights and the vast expanse that was a football field, a narrow corridor formed by beige walls decorated with pictures of doctors and nurses. A woman dressed in white hurried in front of him. She turned and shouted. *Hurry, Paul. This way.*

She walked so fast, Paul needed to run to keep up. He jogged, ran and then sprinted, but failed to keep pace. When the hospital corridor ended at a tee, Paul looked to the left and right, in search of his guide, but the halls were empty, except for gurneys with sheets pulled over motionless bodies that lined the passageway. When he turned to the left and began walking to an open door, the fast nurse reappeared and waved Paul into a room near the end of the hall. The nurse pointed to a gurney, peeled the sheet back revealing Paul's Dad's face and said, *I thought you'd want to say Goodbye.*

Paul's knees buckled and he dropped to the tile floor. Kneeling, he prayed for his Father's soul and picked up a penny that stood on edge, beneath the gurney. He stood, looked into his Dad's closed eyes and apologized. *Sorry I wasn't a football player. Sorry I wouldn't take chances and open my eyes under water, in the ocean, without a bribe. Sorry I wasn't the son you asked for. I tried.*

When Paul's Dad opened his eyes, bolted upright and said, *Too late*, Paul opened his eyes and discovered he was still in a hospital, but not the one where his Dad died, but the one constructed in his home, the one in which he would die. He was in his bedroom, in a bed with siderails, in hospice.

Paul rang the bell that rested on the bed-side table and Mary walked into the room. She smiled. "Did you have a nice nap?"

Paul looked for vestiges of high school football and the beach in the room, and when he saw none, he answered. "It was weird. Vivid dreams."

"The Doctor said the pain medication would cause that. Nightmares?"

"No. Just weird."

Mary clutched the bed rails, adjusted Paul's bed-shirt and asked, "Need anything?"

Paul hadn't heard the question. A part of him remained on Goodrich Field and the beach bordered with oceans of dogs. "Was I a good son? Do you think my Dad loved me?"

"Of course, he did. Why do you ask?"

"I don't know. He wanted a football player, a strapping, daring, kid. I wasn't a football player or very strapping. I was smart, maybe too smart for him. I think he would have traded my brains for more courage. He wanted a boxer, not a student, a stud, not a lawyer. I wonder if I let him down."

"None of us measure up to the ideals we think others have set for us. Your Dad may have been fascinated by rough and tumble boys, he may have dreamed of you in a Green Bay Packers' uniform, but he learned to love you as you were. I have no doubt."

"But he bought me an electric razor when I was in sixth grade. I didn't use it until I was in law school. Didn't have to. He bought me a weight bench and barbells and four years after he bought them, we donated all of it to the Salvation Army, still in the box. He begged me to go out for the high school football team and when I told him I was too small and had no interest, he hung his head. He told me to fight back if a bully bullied me, but when one did, I told the Principal and when she called my dad to meet with him at the school, he was disappointed that I hadn't taken care of it on my own. He wasn't mad at the kid who pushed and taunted me; he was mad at me. He got his hands dirty and expected that every real man would. My hands are clean now and were when he was alive. I think I was a disappointment to him."

Mary brushed the delinquent strand of hair from Paul's forehead, held his hand and waited for it to pass. It always did. The conversation was not new; it had taken place dozens of times during their marriage. When Paul's Dad died, Paul stopped mid-sentence, looked at the coffin in which his Father laid motionless and finished the eulogy with, *Dad, I hope I made you proud, and if not, I'm sorry.* When his Mother died, years after Paul's Dad was buried, Paul asked, *I wonder if she'll convince him that I was a good son?* After a jury trial that ended with an acquittal for a man accused of murder, a man whose innocence Paul doubted, a man Paul defended with creativity and deftness, Paul arrived home after receiving congratulations from his client, his family, the Judge, jurors and the Prosecutor and asked Mary, *I wonder if my dad would've appreciated what I did in the courtroom today?*

Mary didn't have the definitive answer. By the time she met Paul, his dad's business was bankrupt and his dad broken, sullen and silent. She was never able to answer Paul's doubt with memories of what he said or did. She never heard his dad tell Paul, *I love you*, never saw him hug Paul or explain to another that he was proud of his son. She didn't know if he measured up, but knew he should have. He was kind, smart, educated, successful, an exemplary husband and father and a good lawyer. If he wasn't proud, it wasn't Paul's fault; it was the fault of a broken man with unreasonable expectations.

"You haven't disappointed anyone. You're a good man. Any father would be proud to call you son."

After two minutes of silence, it passed. He grinned and spoke. "If I wasn't good enough, Fuck him."

Mary blushed. Even at 74, certain words embarrassed her. *Fuck* was one of those words and when it was spoken, even by her husband, who said it more than Mary wanted, she blushed. "Yes. Fuck him." The blush darkened from pink to red.

"Want me to send in Lauren?"

"Sure. If I can no longer be the good son, maybe I'll try to be the good father."

Lauren walked into Paul's room wearing tennis shorts, tennis shoes and t-shirt that read *USTA Team Tennis*. She stopped when she reached Paul's bed and said, "I'm on my way to a tennis match and thought I'd stop and say *Hi*."

"Hi. I wish I could go and watch. I always enjoyed watching."

"I'll take notes and let you know."

"Lauren, you're a good kid. I'm proud of you."

Confused, Lauren smiled and asked, "Where'd that come from?"

"Nowhere. I just want you to know. And if something happens before I see Alyson and Randy, would you please tell them that I'm proud of them as well."

"I'll tell them, but you'll do so yourself. If I tell them, I'll say you were *almost* as proud of them as me. But, nonetheless, you were proud of them."

"Thanks. Play well and have fun. I'll wait for the report."

Lauren moved the stubborn strand of hair from her Dad's forehead, kissed the hairless brow and walked away. As she was about to leave the room, she turned, grinned and said, "And for what it's worth, you're a great dad and I'm very proud of you."

Paul closed his eyes and slept. The puppies were gone, the football field non-existent. His dad walked to him, smiled, offered his outstretched hand, patted him on the back and said, *Good job, son.*

chapter twelve

When Paul opened his eyes, he saw Belle's face just above his. She was shouting and holding something in her right hand and waving it like a magic wand. It looked like a turkey baster and was filled with what appeared to be red mud. Paul coughed, expelling a red, rubbery mass and took a deep breath. He wasn't running, wasn't playing tennis, wasn't on the mat wrestling with another eighth grader, yet he was breathless and needed to continue to gulp air and draw it deep into his cancer ravaged lungs. After Paul took eight deep breaths, Belle straightened her back, moving her face from near Paul's and set the baster on the bedside table.

Belle wiped sweat from Paul's forehead, and with the same tissue, wiped sweat from her brow. She smiled and spoke. "Thought we lost you."

Paul narrowed his eyes. He was skeptical. Had he nearly slept through his own death? *Nah.* "Huh?"

"Some stuff got stuck in your throat. You couldn't breathe. When I came in you were trying to draw in air, but couldn't. Your mouth was open and you were trying, but getting nowhere. I looked down your throat, which you presented perfectly, saw an obstruction and suctioned it out." Belle smiled and chuckled. "And sir, after I did all the skill work, you opened your eyes and breathed."

"I had no idea. I opened my eyes, saw you and your magic wand and sucked in air. I almost missed it."

Belle put her hands on her hips, drew in some air that Paul had left in the room, grinned, exhaled with exuberance and shook her head.

"Thank you, Belle. I think you saved my life. You and your magic wand."

Belle blushed, looked to the heavens and accepted the praise. "I suppose I did. But, that's why I'm here. It's my job. You're in hospice, so efforts to save you from cancer have been terminated, but if something else appears and makes you uncomfortable or vulnerable and I can remove it, I will. And I did. Glad I could." She looked at her hands which were trembling and lifted them so Paul could see. "Don't do it again. I'm not sure I could control the magic wand again."

Belle lifted the bell and shook it, calling for Mary. Before Mary walked through the door, Paul asked Belle to come close and when she did, he whispered, "Our secret. When I'm gone, you explain what just happened, but not now. No need in making Mary and the kids more nervous than they already are."

Belle drew an imaginary key from her pocket and locked her mouth shut. She winked and as Mary approached the bed, she made a circle from her thumb and index finger, and waved it in front of Paul's eyes. Mary saw and wondered, "Okay what?"

Belle left the bedside for the doorway, grinned at Paul and maintained her commitment to secrecy. She hid the wand filled with blood and sludge behind her back, inched in reverse toward the door, winked and said, "Never you mind."

"Sleep well?"

"I thought so. Pleasant dreams." Paul reached for his wife's left hand, which rested on the bedrail. She wore the ring Paul had given her almost a half-century earlier.

Paul didn't think she had removed the ring since she he slid it on her finger in 1968. It was always there. When she gave birth to their children and had minor surgery, doctors suggested she place it in a plastic bag for safekeeping, but she chose to wrap it in cotton strips held in place by medical tape. When she swam, Paul was afraid it would fall to the bottom of the lake, but Mary said, *Don't worry. I swim with my left hand in a fist. Slows me down, but keeps the ring in place.* When she turned 40 and added pounds, the ring pinched her finger, making it look like a long, slender balloon, tied in the middle. Paul suggested she remove it so that she didn't damage her finger with obstructed circulation, but she disagreed and said, *If my finger turns black, I'll do it, but until then, No.* When she celebrated her seventieth birthday, when pounds were difficult to maintain and her fingers more slender than ever before, Paul was concerned the ring would slip from the skinny digit and suggested she remove it, so it could be sized and remain snug on her finger. Mary said *No*, found a jeweler who was willing to attach a spacer to the ring while it remained on Mary's finger, and kept it on.

Paul rotated the ring on Mary's finger so that the stone faced the ceiling. "Will you ever take it off?"

The question asked begged for an explanation, prose dedicated to love and commitment. Always concise, Mary answered with, "Nope." She stuck her tongue out of her mouth, lifted the corners of her mouth and said no more.

"Do you remember the day I put it on your finger?"

"May 30, 1968. 7:00 p.m. We were at Law's Barbeque, sitting in a booth under a *Schlitz* sign. The tablecloth was plastic and red-checked. You wore a gray sweatshirt, blue jeans and cowboy boots. When I think about it, it's the only time I've ever seen you in cowboy boots. But, on that day you wore them. Maybe you were trying to add some inches, improve our chances. You ordered a pulled pork sandwich, French fries, and in honor of the sign, a Schlitz. After Dan refilled your beer glass, you reached in your pocket, set in on the plastic tablecloth and asked, *Will you marry me?* I said *Yes,* you slid the ring on my finger and it's still there. They'll bury me with it on." She smiled and laughed. "And, No, I don't remember."

"You have two daughters. Maybe one would like to have Mom's ring."

"Call me selfish. It's mine, just mine. I'll die with it on my finger, believing it'll be buried with me. If one of them slips it from my finger after I'm dead, so be it. They have our mothers' rings; they don't need mine."

"Can I hold it in my hand? Wrap my hand around it?"

"Nope. It isn't coming off my finger. Sorry. You gave it to me and I'm keeping it."

"What if long after I'm gone, Rex proposes and you accept?"

Mary grinned at the thought of her old neighbor, a widower for years, a troll for life, asking her to marry him. She'd rather die alone, or marry mutton, before the slaughter, but humored her husband. He was dying, bed ridden and in need of humor. "Rex? Your ring would be in the trash the next day."

Paul gurgled. Six months ago, it would have been a chuckle. On that day, it was a smiling gurgle. "My ass. That fucker."

Mary blushed. "Watch your language old man. I'll get a bar of soap. You're not too old for correction."

Paul smiled. She was right. He had been coarse and needed to moderate his language. Although her demand was accompanied by a smile, she deserved what she had asked for. Mary was raised by a drunken, mentally ill woman, whose personal struggles made it impossible for her to tend to her daughter. Mary received little direction, almost no correction, yet she developed into a good and honest young woman, and when called upon, a marvelous mother. She had no training, no example, but she excelled at her craft. As Paul laid dying, recognizing they'd never again dance, travel or make love, looking at his wife, marveling in her goodness, he understood, he was a lucky man.

Paul often asked Mary if his Dad loved him, accepted him, was proud of him; Mary had no similar concerns. Mary didn't wonder if her mother loved her or was proud of her, she worried she might become her.

At an office Christmas party in 1980, a junior law partner asked Mary if she wanted a drink and she answered, *No, I don't drink.* In 1990, when that junior partner had become a senior partner, he asked Mary if he could get her a drink and she said, *Sorry, I don't drink.* Much later that evening, when the senior partner had consumed enough alcohol for Mary and him, when his reticence had been swallowed by vodka and his reluctance had been drowned by gin, with confidence and impetuousness fueled by booze, he sat next to Mary and asked, *Why not? Why don't you party with us?* In spite of the offensive question and boorish conduct, Mary smiled at her drunken interviewer and whispered in his ear, *Because unlike you, I don't want to become an embarrassment.*

Paul knew. The answer was clear. He and Mary had discussed it often. The discussion began in 1967, in a courtroom, while Mary sat in the witness stand and her mother sat next to Paul.

Paul enlightened his drunken co-worker, at the office, the next day, when he was sober. He walked into his office unannounced, stood over his desk, looked into his blood-shot eyes and spoke quietly, so as not to disturb what was likely a pounding head. *Mary doesn't drink because she's witnessed its devastation.*

Please, don't ask her again. Before Paul's surprised co-worker could ask why the message was given to him, before he could defend himself by saying he hadn't asked, in fuzzy shades of gray, he remembered, so he simply smiled, nodded his head and returned to the papers on his desk.

Genetics haunted Mary. When the homeless shelter where Mary worked taxed her energies while her own children made impossible demands of her time, she slept later than usual and when she rose from bed asked, *Do you think I'm suffering from depression, staying in bed when I should be up and productive?* When her gall bladder was breaking, she was unable to sleep and when up and about, clutched her belly and complained about discomfort. When her doctor was unable to discern the cause of her bellyache, she asked Paul, *Am I imagining this, am I a hypochondriac or worse, schizophrenic?*

Mary's mother was dead, but she was ever present in Mary's fears. *Like mother, like daughter.* She read books about genetics, heredity, mental illness. She said the books helped her understand the population the shelter served, helped her at work; Paul suspected they helped her at home, while in bed, consumed by worry, helped her understand her mother and herself.

Genetics haunted Mary; they never infected her. Paul didn't know anyone more stable. She was sane, sober and happy. And she loved Paul.

Paul patted the hand that wore a diamond gifted 47 years before and asked, "Do you want to dance?"

Mary smiled and extended her right hand, asking Paul to take it in his left and lead. She closed her eyes as Paul closed his, and they danced. They were old, feeble, unable to tap the floor, but with their eyes closed and their imaginations active, they danced, elegantly, seductively, beautifully. When the music stopped, Paul opened his eyes, looked into the green eyes of his sane and sober lover, cleared his throat, winked, smiled and whispered, "I am now, and over the last 48 years, have been, a very lucky man. Thank you."

chapter thirteen

Paul was tired. His legs ached and he was winded. His dancing shoes were tight; pinching his long toes together and suppressing his arch. He found an imaginary bench, waltzed to it, sat and rested his legs and removed his shoes, so he could massage the pain from his feet. Supine on his bed, locked in by side-rails and a body crippled by cancer, Paul imagined bare feet and the relief for which his dancing feet cried. He couldn't leave his bed, but he could dream and in his dreams, dance, tire, ache and reduce the pain by lifting tired feet from the dance floor, expose them and massage.

Paul looked at Mary, whose hand remained in his, exhaled, drew in a deep breath, softly chuckled and said, "I'm not as young as I once was. That dancing took it out of me."

With her free hand, Mary tapped the top of the hand that held hers, smiled and said, "You were marvelous. I had a hard time keeping up. You are as good a dancer as that man I married 47-years ago. My feet hurt. Damn you're good."

Paul was on a roll, doing in his mind, what his body had forbidden months ago. He couldn't leap from his bed, at least not literally, but he could close his eyes and fly, soar to places unseen. He'd danced with his bride without leaving his bed and wondered what else he could do. *Run a three-minute mile? Win the U.S. Open, beating Federer in three sets? Convince the Supreme Court to reverse the murder conviction of a young innocent man who was prosecuted because he was brown and convenient? Ride a gentle, but large, white horse through a gorge between majestic mountains? Or....?* He grinned a prurient grin, leered at his 73 year old wife, and drooled. He closed his eyes, drew her near, pealed the clothes from her body, took her in his arms and three minutes later opened his eyes, exhausted, spent, satisfied.

Still holding Mary's hand in his, Paul wiped sweat from his brow with his free hand, blushed and softly ended the sexual encounter. "That was good. Who's next?"

Mary ignored the question and asked about the statement. "What was good?"

Paul withdrew his hand from Mary's, placed a fictional cigarette in his mouth and lit it with an imaginary match. He blew non-existent smoke into the air and answered Mary's question. "A cigarette always tastes so good after intimacy."

Mary stood, erased wrinkles in her ravaged clothing with palms acting as irons, blushed and asked, "Was it good?"

Paul didn't speak; he didn't have to. His broad smile was as articulate as words.

When Mary reached the doorway, she turned, adjusted her underwear and bra and coiffed her hair with fingers and asked her lover, "Do I look okay? Does it show?"

"They'll never know."

Two minutes after Mary disappeared, Ron Scott walked through the door with a broad smile. As soon as he knew Paul was awake and his enthusiasm wouldn't wake him, Ron melodically said, "My friend, how are you?"

Ron was musical. He didn't play an instrument, wasn't a singer making records or a conductor waving a wand, but he was a musician. He spoke in rhythms and melodies. His voice was deep, resonate, clear. Ron's music wasn't intentional; his sentences weren't lyrics sets to a tune. He wasn't Joel Gray in *Cabaret*, Fred Astaire in *Holiday Inn* or Gene Kelly in *Singing in the Rain*; he was simply Ron Scott, living what he considered a good and blessed life, a life with syncopation, notes played by an in-tune tuba, arias, acoustic guitars and refrains. He was always happy, always upbeat, positive, optimistic, grateful and on-key. His glee was reflected in his ever-smiling face and the lilt and melody in his voice.

And, his joy was contagious. Paul, tired from dance and sex, imaginary as they were, opened his eyes wide and felt the corners of his mouth reach for the clear, blue, sky of Ron's world. "I'm alive. And you?"

"Wonderful. No regrets, no obstacles to happiness. In large part, because of you."

Paul had helped. He knew Ron's life would have been different, but for Paul, but Paul was humble, unwilling to publicly accept responsibility. "I played only a minor role Ron. Your life is what it is, because it's the way you chose to live it."

"You are too kind and humble, my friend."

Paul tried to identify the musical group who had performed *You Are Too Humble and Kind My Friend*. The song was familiar, the lyric enlightening, the melody catchy. Ron covered the song with aplomb. Paul believed he would fall asleep later that afternoon, with the tune resonating in his addled brain. *You Are Too Humble and Kind My Friend*. Ron Scott, the unintended musician.

"What's new in your life, Ron?"

"Nothing significant. I'm staying on course, doing what needs to be done and reaping the rewards. How about you? How are you feeling?"

"Not bad for a dying man. I think I've mastered dying. Kill the pain with drugs, reminisce with old friends, deny the inevitability of the end and dream. I soar to places unseen. There's always hope. Not for another decade or another year, but for a chance for happiness, no matter how long it lasts."

"You have always been wise." *Elvis? Elton John? Sinatra?*

Ron looked at the bedside chair, asked for permission to sit with the palms of his outstretched hands, received it and sat. "I hope

I will still be visiting with you years from now, here or on the town, but we never know, so felt the need to get here today and thank you one more time." *Elvis singing Gospel.*

"You've thanked me too many times, Ron. No need for further thanks. You built me a retaining wall out back, took my kids to church and hockey when we couldn't, drove me to the doctor when Mary was sick and have been a good, reliable, generous friend. Further thanks are unnecessary."

"I know, but thanking you reminds me of what could have been and helps me continue to appreciate what I have. Thank you again, my friend."

"It wasn't just me."

Paul didn't believe in divine intervention; he believed it had all been set in motion and the creator that set it in motion, watched, but didn't interfere. When football teams won the big game and the game's star thanked God for his role in the victory, Paul wondered if that meant God had determined the losing team unworthy of victory. When doctors healed children with cancer and parents thanked not medicine but God for the child's recovery, Paul wondered if that meant God had infected the child with cancer in the first place and if the doctors' efforts were irrelevant. Paul didn't deny the existence of God. He was a good, but skeptical Lutheran, and celebrated God's existence, but was unwilling to assign responsibility for all good and bad, to God. He made an exception in Ron's case.

Ron asked, "If not you, who?"

"Divine intervention. I don't know. Not me."

Paul had never been able to explain it. It was real, unlike imaginary sex. It had happened, unlike an imaginary dance between a bed-ridden, dying man and his willing and able partner. It had happened and was real.

Two children from Iowa were found dead in St. Cloud, Minnesota. The children's bodies were mutilated and medical examiners discovered they had been sexually assaulted.

The murdered Iowans were found in 1990, while Jacob Wetterling, a child abducted from Central Minnesota in 1989, remained missing. The Wetterling case consumed Minnesota. Jacob was with two friends, not far from home, when a man confronted the three, took Jacob and disappeared. The County investigated, the State investigated, the Feds investigated. All three were unsuccessful. Jacob's whereabouts were unknown, his fate, an unanswered riddle. The public was fascinated by the case and hungered for answers and justice.

As the public clamored for answers to Jacob's abduction, two children near Jacob's age, were found dead twenty miles from Jacob's home. When a man was arrested for the murders, it was the answer the passionate, yet uneducated masses, wanted. Almost everyone believed the accused not only killed the two children from Iowa found in a mucky swamp; they believed he had killed Jacob Wetterling.

Ron Scott was the accused, the most hated man in Minnesota.

Ron lived in Clearwater, two minutes from where the bodies were found. People who lived near where the bodies were discovered, described an unfamiliar car that had been in their neighborhood days before the victims were found and police made impressions of tire tracks found near the swamp. When a witness told the police, he had seen a car similar to the one that he saw near the swamp, abandoned on Sherburne County Road 16, the investigators found it and after receiving permission from its owner, searched it and found blood and burial tools in the trunk. Ron was the car's registered owner.

Before Ron was questioned by the police, before he was detained, the St. Cloud Times learned that Ron was a person of interest, and given the public's intense interest in the case and the Wetterling case, and its desire to sell subscriptions, it ignored the law and ran a story suggesting the police had identified the killer of two children from Iowa and perhaps Jacob Wetterling, Ron Scott. Before he was questioned, Ron had been convicted by the press and anyone who read a newspaper or watched a television. Everyone.

Ron denied involvement, but when investigators found blood on the door to Ron's apartment, when a search consistent with a warrant discovered boots in Ron's closet that were caked with mud that resembled the mud of the swamp where the bodies of the children were found, when his estranged spouse who was a bit off-kilter and stung by divorce papers, told investigators that Ron had a thing for kids and when they were unable to confirm his alibi, he was charged with two counts of murder.

The public had heard enough. In coffee shops, work breakrooms and on the telephone, he wasn't referred to as the accused, but rather, *the fucker who killed Jacob Wetterling*. Classmates Ron hadn't seen in a decade, remembered him as shifty and a little too interested in their younger siblings. Ron's neighbors described him as a loner, around whom they'd never felt comfortable. Talk-show hosts suggested Ron be tortured to the extent necessary to pry a confession and location of Jacob Wetterling's body, and then executed.

The Wright County Attorney convened a grand jury to consider the case and hopefully, obtain indictments for first degree murder, but while the grand jury questioned investigators, the federal government charged Ron with two counts of capital murder, alleging he had transported the children across state lines, making it a federal crime subject to the death penalty. Relieved of responsibility, the Wright County Attorney smiled. Believing Ron would soon be killed for his despicable deeds, the public cheered. Understanding he was likely done, that his freedom had disappeared and his life would soon end, Ron cried.

Ron was condemned, convicted without a trial. Everyone believed he was guilty and that a trial was an unnecessary waste of time and money. As the *Patriot* announcer said into his microphone and to thousands of listeners, *Kill him and be done with it.*

Ron was being held in the Sherburne County Jail, which housed federal prisoners for a price. The *Star News*, Elk River's local newspaper ran a story about the killer held in its midst. The reporter traveled to the Courthouse, which was connected to the jail, and asked locals how they felt about the killer in their community. Most said they were afraid, angry and hoped the execution would take place soon so they could return to their quiet, safe, comfortable lives. Paul was questioned by the *Star News* reporter and gave a different answer. His answer was printed in full, and attributed to Paul Thomas, a local lawyer.

I'm in no mood to condemn this guy. If he did it, damn him. If he did it, may he rot in Hell after he is convicted by a jury and executed by the authorities. But, I'm not so sure he did it. He denies it, claims the evidence is inconclusive. Everyone has concluded he not only killed two kids from Iowa, but that he killed Jacob Wetterling. They've reached that conclusion based on not very much. They've reached that conclusion, because they want a conclusion, a responsible party, someone to blame and punish. Let the system do what it was intended to do. Let the Federal Government prove its case in Court and when it does, ask me if I think he should die, and I will likely say yes. But, until then, while he is shielded by the law, which says everyone, including Ron Scott, is presumed innocent until proved guilty beyond a reasonable doubt, don't ask me to condemn him. Shame on you for asking.

Ten days after the story appeared in the *Star News*, Paul was patched into a telephone conference call that included a federal district court judge and the man prosecuting Ron Scott.

"Mr. Thomas, thank you for taking my call. This is Judge Douglas."

"Good morning your honor." Paul stood, stretched the chord that connected the handpiece to the phone base, and closed his office door.

"I have Rick Brown on the line. Rick, are you still here?"

"I am. Good morning, Mr. Thomas."

Paul didn't know Rick Brown, but had seen him on television, pleading with the reporters to let him do his job. *Don't forget, he's not been convicted, and until he is, he is an innocent man. Please remember that.*

"Mr. Brown."

"Mr. Thomas, Mr. Brown and I have a problem and maybe you can help."

Afraid of what was to be said, but maintaining respect for a federal judge with immense power and a lifetime appointment, Paul answered with statement followed by a question. "I'm always willing to help a fellow traveler. How can I help?"

"I'll be blunt. I need to find someone to represent Ron Scott. He's broke, so can't afford to hire a lawyer. The Public Defenders' Office has claimed a conflict, something related to Jacob Wetterling and our conflict lawyers, all in private practice, refuse to accept representation, believing that if they did, their private practices will be destroyed."

"But, I'm in private practice. Why would you believe I'm willing to jeopardize my practice by representing Scott?"

The Judge cleared his throat and gave the answer Paul knew he would receive. "Because, you've already jeopardized your practice. When you told the press that Ron Scott was innocent until proven guilty, you took a stand, showed courage and jeopardized your practice. You're the only person with nothing left to lose."

"But, I haven't tried a criminal case in years and never in federal court."

The Judge was skilled. He had anticipated the obstacles and had answers for them. "I've talked to Judge Coyne and Judge Meyer, they both said you were beyond competent. Brilliant is the word they both used. According to each, you tried cases before them and did a great job. And the Federal system is not so different than the State. If you accept, we will appoint a federal prosecutor from out-of-state, to work with you. You'd be in charge, it's your voice the jurors would hear, he'd simply keep you out of trouble when it came to Federal Rules."

Paul's chest swelled. *Brilliant? Judge Coyne and Judge Meyer? Brilliant? Probably not, but brilliant?*

They talked about compensation, duration and location. Paul had all of the information he needed to make a decision.

It was hard to tell a Federal Judge *No*, so Paul tried to end the conversation with, "Let me think about it, and talk to my partners and my wife. It's a big commitment."

The Judge had anticipated the conference call would end as Paul had attempted to end it. He had a couple of things to add. "Understood. Discuss it and get back to my clerk. And please be quick. The system moves quickly and Mr. Scott is entitled to good and competent representation."

Paul formed the words *Good Bye* in his mind and was about to utter them, when the Judge added a thought. "And Mr. Thomas, maybe you could meet with Mr. Scott before you make a decision. I can provide you with access, without requiring you to come on board. I never could have represented my mother; my dad would have been a dream client. I don't expect you can make a decision before you determine if Mr. Scott is my mom or dad."

"I'm sure he's neither, Your Honor, but understand. I will do what I can, as quickly as I can. Thanks for the honor of being asked."

After talking to partners and Mary, Paul learned they were fascinated by their proximity to the headlines. *We can cover for you here. The kids and I will be fine if you're distracted and gone for a while.* In unison. *Go for it.*

The next morning, Paul walked to the front desk of the Sherburne County jail and before he could identify himself, the desk clerk hit a button, opened a secure door and asked Paul to wait around the corner while jailers brought Mr. Scott to the interview area.

Paul expected Ron would nauseate him. He anticipated he would be, slimy, degenerate, shifty, prurient, guilty. He was surprised.

Ron was respectful, polite, humble, quiet, unless asked to be otherwise, and kind. He understood the gravity of his condition, knew he was facing a death sentence and a substantial amount of damaging evidence, but convincingly claimed innocence.

When Paul asked Ron why there was blood on his apartment doorknob, Ron said, "I don't know?" When he was asked why his trunk was littered with blood and burial equipment, he said, "I don't know." He explained why his estranged wife would lie and make false accusations, but had no explanation for why the boots in his closet were caked with mud that was similar to the mud in the swamp were the children's bodies were found. His answers were incomplete, evasive, self-serving, and yet, Paul believed him.

Ron didn't speak, he sang. No tunes, no refrains, music. The music that was his voice was convincing. When Ron spoke, Paul found his foot tapping to the words, keeping the beat. He was washed and moved by the music. Paul had prosecuted conmen, defended criminals who dishonestly explained their guilt away with convincing words. He had been to war with consummate liars and knew people would say and do anything for money, let alone for their lives, so he was skeptical. Paul's experience as a prosecutor and public defender dashed his Pollyannaish naivety and filled his soul with cynicism. But, the weather-beaten cynic believed Ron. His aria was convincing.

Paul represented Ron.

Rick Brown was an impersonal adversary, the Judge, no longer a salesman, a tyrant, proving to the press and those who read or watched, that he had little time or sympathies for a man who killed three children.

Always interested in an agreement that would avoid a jury trial, Paul negotiated with Rick, to no avail. Rick's best offer asked Ron to plead guilty to one count of murder and let the Judge sentence as the Judge saw fit. Ron was consistent in his claim of innocence and both he and Paul knew that the Prosecutor's offer was an invitation to death by lethal injection, so it was rejected. Without a reasonable alternative, the case proceeded to trial.

The Government's evidence was extensive and pointed to Ron as the killer of two innocent children from Iowa, and Ron had no explanation for its existence, so Paul decided that he would defend Ron by arguing that mud is mud, blood is blood, a car was stolen and that Ron was in Ft. Leavenworth, Kansas, serving his country, when Jacob Wetterling was abducted. Ron was not charged with Jacob's kidnapping, but everyone assumed he had kidnapped and killed Jacob, and Paul believed if he could show Ron had not done one of the things the public believed he had done, kidnap and kill Jacob Wetterling, the jury might question the Government's case against Ron and find it had not proven the allegations beyond a reasonable doubt.

The Government's Agronomist testified that the mud found on Ron's boots matched mud taken from the swamp where the children's bodies had been buried. When Paul asked if other swamps in other places might have mud that matched the mud on Ron's boots and the swamp where the victims were found, he said, *Yes*.

The Government's Medical Examiner testified that blood found in Ron's car's trunk and on his doorknob, was similar to the victim's blood, but admitted that millions of other people have similar blood, including perhaps, Ron's neighbor or landlord.

Before the Government rested, it recalled its lead investigator. As he took the stand, he held a quart-sized paper bag that contained something small and light. When questioned by Brown, he removed a hat from the bag and testified that it was found in the trunk of Ron's car and that the children's grieving mother had identified it as a hat she had given her son, three days before he was found buried in mud.

Seemingly, as an afterthought, Brown asked the witness, if mud was mud, why did he believe Ron Scott's boots were worn by the killer and he said for the first time, that he had observed boot prints in the mud, baked in place by the sun, and those prints mirrored the pattern in the boots found at Ron Brown's home.

Paul objected to the testimony and the introduction of the hat as evidence, claiming it hadn't been previously disclosed, and as a result should not be admitted, but after Brown argued it was rebuttal evidence not subject to the same disclosure rules as substantive evidence, Douglas overruled the objection, and seemingly convicted Ron.

Paul called one witness, Ron. His direct testimony was short. He sang. The song was beautiful. Melodically he said his car was stolen and abandoned on a county road, that he had no idea how blood was applied to his doorknob or deposited in his trunk, that his estranged spouse's imperfect mental health had led to divorce papers and when she received them, vowed, *to get you, you son-of-a-bitch*, that he'd never seen the child's hat and that he often wore boots when it was wet and muddy.

Paul walked to the witness stand, smiled at his client who made music without notes, and asked, "Do you remember October 22, 1989?"

"Yes, I do."

"Why is that date memorable?"

"That's the day Jacob Wetterling was abducted."

"Where were you on that day?"

"I was a soldier stationed at Ft. Leonard Wood, Kentucky."

"And why is it you remember where you were on that day?"

"I was sent to South Korea the next day. On October 22, 1989, I packed with the rest of my squadron and the next day, October 23, 1989, we boarded a plane and flew to South Korea."

"Thank you for your service Mr. Scott. No more questions."

Rick Brown cross-examined Ron for two hours. It was exercise in futility. Those who lie are oftentimes caught in their lies. People who misperceive, are often caught in their misperceptions. People who remember things vividly, those who describe every detail of an ancient occurrence, often are caught in faulty memories. Ron didn't lie, didn't explain what couldn't be explained and provided no details, just a denial and an absolute alibi to the disappearance of Jacob Wetterling, so try as he might, Rick Brown made no points during his cross-examination of Ron. Ron's music was compelling, convincing.

Three jurors cried when Rick Brown made his final argument. He spoke softly, slowly. He pointed at pictures of dead children and pointed at Ron, accusing him of unthinkable acts. He listed items of evidence introduced and reasoned that the evidence's existence and location meant only one thing, that Ron Scott had acted on a sexual impulse and killed two children.

When Brown completed his argument, and sat in his chair, everyone looked to Paul. He was next to perform and all were anxious to hear what he had to say. Paul sat silently in his chair. He was still, quiet. He looked at his notes, but didn't scribble. He sat, still, quiet.

Judge Douglas asked, *Mr. Thomas?*, but Paul didn't answer, and instead remained seated, saying nothing. When the silence was uncomfortable, when it eclipsed Brown's final argument, when the jurors forgot what had been said and were wondering what would be said, Paul stood.

Paul talked about reasonable, alternative explanations and the Prosecutor's burden to prove guilt, *beyond a reasonable doubt*, but he focused on music. He couldn't sing like Ron had, couldn't bring melody to the defense as Ron had, but wanted to remind the jury that music is magical and good, and hoped they had appreciated the beautiful performance Ron's orchestra had given. He exhibited a goodness, an innocence, a melodic answer to evil and Paul reminded them of the song they had heard. Ron had convinced Paul months earlier, not with evidence or explanations, but with music. Paul hoped the jurors weren't tone deaf, that they had heard and believed.

"Ladies and gentlemen, evil still lurks. It's out there and it's my hope that the investigators who wrongfully concluded Ron Scott was evil, hear the music, recognize Mr. Scott's innocence and find the person responsible for the death of two children. Thank you."

Four days after the jury began its deliberations, it found Ron Scott not guilty of all counts. Five weeks after Ron was released from custody, a grifter in North Dakota confessed to kidnapping and killing two children from Iowa, and stealing a car in Clearwater, Minnesota. He drove investigators to the swamp where the children were found and found his abandoned car off a dirt-road in Santiago Township. His car's exterior was covered in dust and its interior covered in blood. He pleaded guilty to kidnapping and murder and asked the Court to execute him and end his sexual and murderous nightmare. He was convicted and sentenced to death. Eight years after the jury freed Ron Scott, a doctor injected the confessed killer and he died.

Paul pushed a button and his bed lifted him so he could look into the eyes of his acquitted friend. "Divine intervention, my friend. Something converted your words to music and made them believable. It wasn't me. I helped. You helped, but something turned an alibi into a song, an explanation into a melody and a defense into a concert. Never before, never since."

"I think you're right. The song remains. It's why I'm happy. It's why I'm positive, upbeat and optimistic. The tune plays over and over. It's sweet, innocent, refreshing and beautiful. It saved me and guides me."

Ron stood, hummed, smiled, took hold of the bedrails and after an uncomfortable silence that shifted Paul's focus from what had been said to what would be said, made his final argument. "But, what you don't ever seem to understand is, you're the orchestra leader, the composer. Without you, there'd have been no aria, no symphony and if not, I'd have been convicted and North

Dakota cops would have never questioned the killer about the killing. I'd have been put to death. Without you."

Paul closed his eyes and silently accepted responsibility. He tapped an imaginary lectern with an imaginary baton, listened as instruments were lifted from laps and held in the ready position, waited for the music and smiled.

"Thanks, Ron. I'm glad it worked out. Maybe in a week or two, I can thank the responsible party."

Ron took Paul's hand in his, squeezed gently and said, "I already have and will again. Thank you, my friend."

Paul didn't see Ron leave the room. After imaginary sex, a pretend dance and a murder trial in federal court, Paul was tired, and when he attempted to blink, his eyes remained closed, and exhausted, he slept.

Ron stood at a microphone in the middle of a large stadium. He spoke and the crowd cheered. He strummed a guitar he held, but the guitar didn't play notes or musical chords, it sounded words that Ron had spoken during his glee-filled life. A back-up singer leaned into the microphone, opened his mouth and with a tambourine in hand, pleaded for leniency, the words and voice not his, but Ron's. As Ron left the stage, the audience rose to its collective feet and applauded, screaming for an encore. Ron reappeared, asked the crowd to sit, nodded *Yes* to their request for an encore, pulled the microphone close, and after an uncomfortable silence so long the audience forgot what preceded it, said, sang, whistled, *Ladies and gentlemen, evil still lurks. It's out there and it's my hope that the investigators who wrongfully concluded Ron Scott was evil, hear the music, recognize Mr. Scott's innocence and find the person responsible for the death of two children. Thank you.*

chapter fourteen

Paul wasn't certain if he was awake or still asleep. When he opened his eyes, Frank Nistler stood before him with an iPad in hand. He was poised to hit a button and show Paul something on his device's small screen. His smile was broad, his anticipation great, almost cartoon-like. He stood still, waiting. It was as if Frank had been paused by a button. He stood, he waited, he anxiously anticipated that the button would be depressed and he could return to action and bring life to himself and his iPad's screen. He waited, motionless. Paul wasn't sure if Frank was there in his room or in his dream.

Paul wiped sleep from his eyes, focused on the cartoon character who stood before him, silent and still, cleared a throat that couldn't be cleared, gathered his thoughts, concluded he was awake and Frank was real, and spoke. "Frank?"

Frank snapped to action. Paul's word was the button and Frank was freed from his pause, engaged and moving like film moving through the vision gate after a stoppage. "Good! Look at this!"

Frank touched the screen of his iPad and a picture moved across the glass face. Ernie Els stood over a putt, his ball five feet from the cup. The green was surrounded by spectators who silently watched the German draw his putter back and launch the ball toward the hole. When the ball found the cup and fell, the crowd cheered and Frank said to Paul, "Wait, listen, listen…"

The crowd on the screen became quiet as Ernie reached into the cup and removed his ball and held it for the audience, thanking its members for their support. Before the announcers spoke, from a distance, beyond the green, beyond the crowd that circled the green, a voice in an ocean of silence shouted, *You da man, Ernie*, and Frank beamed.

"Did you hear it? Did you hear it?" The 76-year old man in plaid shorts and a tee-shirt that boasted of *Schweaty Meats*, danced on the floor of Paul's hospice and held his iPad over his head in celebration. Very pleased with himself, he asked, "Want to hear it again?"

"No Frank. I heard it clearly." Sarcastically, Paul added, "I watched the tournament on T.V. and thought I heard you then."

Frank's enthusiasm was about to burst his small head that was contained by a thick skull, thin skin and a ball cap that read, *Titleist*. "Did you really hear it *when* I yelled it?"

"No Frank. I didn't hear it. I don't listen for it. I know you'll always find me and play it for me. I'm not hard to find."

Frank graduated high school in 1956, a year before Paul. They lived in the same neighborhood, played on the same baseball and basketball teams, walked to school together and when 16, Paul repeatedly, day-after-day, pushed Frank's '41 Plymouth down the road, so Frank could pop the clutch and start his finicky hardtop, so Frank could drive the two to school. They were friends from second grade, to graduation, to hospice.

Frank joined the Army after graduation and served for 12 years, before receiving a medical discharge. *Bad ears, deficient hearing.* His ear drums were damaged by the constant discharge of the Army's heavy guns, which Frank was required to load. **BOOM BOOM**, became **BOOM BOOM**, became **boom boom** became **boom boom** became **boom boom**.

Frank received disability checks, asked friends to *speak up*, and listened to music so loud, others left the room, some the building.

In 1964, Frank listened to an album recorded live by the Beach Boys. When he turned the record to side 2, turned the volume up, and listened to *Papa-Oom-Mow-Mow,* he heard the crowd and was changed. He called Paul after listening to the album for the first time.

"Paul, have you heard *Beach Boys Concert?*"

Paul was a Beatles' guy, attending law school. Between books, if Paul listened to records, it was Beatles music he heard, not the Beach Boys. He hadn't heard the album and had no interest in ever hearing it. The Beach Boys were American, talented, musical and genius, they just didn't play music Paul enjoyed. He didn't surf, wasn't interested in *Surfer Girl*s or a *Little Deuce*

Coup, so he turned the dial when the Beach Boys' music played and had never purchased a Beach Boys record. "Nope. I've not heard it."

"I think you said No, but I'm not sure. Speak up."

Paul shouted into the mouthpiece. "**No.**"

"Thanks, that's better. I'm listening now. Good music, but what's amazing is the noise of the audience. As the music is being performed and recorded, the audience reacts and their reactions have become part of the recording. I can hear people applauding, encouraging, singing along. They are part of it. They're unnamed collaborators, artists without recognition. It is so cool."

Beach Boys Concert was Frank's invitation, a map of his future. He did what those who were present when *Beach Boys Concert* was recorded had done. He attended, shouted and became a part of the performance.

He attended concerts and in between songs, when it was otherwise quiet, shouted his approval or loudly demanded a favorite track or an encore. He went to basketball games, golf matches and hockey games in empty arenas where his voice would carry, be heard and recorded by television cameras there to entertain its nightly news audience. At baseball games, he hunted home-run balls in the outfield, wearing fluorescent lime green or pink clothing, designed to catch the eye of the camera and public. *If you can't hear me, you can see me.*

Frank had three televisions, three VCR's and an insatiable appetite. He recorded games he attended and the news that reported on them. Thereafter, he listened to his recordings, waiting, hoping to hear himself. And when he did, he was overjoyed, apoplectic, insanely happy to know he was part of it, not just an observer. He listened to himself, over and over. He compiled a master tape of his many recorded outbursts and played it for anyone willing to listen to 1,486 entries of *You da man, Play Your Song, Play Hound Dog, Good goal, The best, Come on Ref, Unbelievable, Minnesota rules, Gophers rule, What a joke, Go Kirby, Go Herbie, Go Gophers, Go Wolves, Go Sioux, You gotta be kidding, McEnroe rules,* and now, *You da man, Ernie.*

"Where was the tournament?"

"Oakmont. CBS was there. Golf Channel did Thursday and Friday, CBS Saturday and Sunday. I got on six times Thursday. No competition. Very few people there, so I had the airwaves to myself. More people on the weekend. I listened to the CBS tapes. I think I was on once on Saturday and maybe twice Sunday. Sometimes it's hard to tell. Too many people doing the same thing. No respect for the experienced. They shout over me. Shit, I was doing this before they were born. I wish they'd shut up and let me get some clear recordings. I have to fight for the stage. Not fair."

"Ungrateful clowns." Paul was attempting sarcasm, poking fun at Frank's hobby, but Frank took what he did seriously and failed to see the humor. He appreciated Paul's words, believing they were sympathetic.

"Nope it isn't. Fairness has evaporated. In the old days, I was alone. No one bothered me. I waited, it got quiet and I'd add something that was recorded and added to the event. No more. I miss the old days."

Frank's head fell forward and his smile disappeared as he longed for the days when he could interrupt quiet anticipation with a childish shout. Melancholic, sad about changes that stole his misplaced thunder, Frank was quiet, still, as if the pause button had been depressed again.

Paul felt sorry for his old friend. His '41 Plymouth wouldn't start, he was unable to retire healthy after 20 years from the Army, couldn't hear life's subtle songs and found pleasure by perverting the professional performances of others. He was incomplete, a puzzle only partially constructed. No family, no employment, no significant contribution, just a compilation of recorded outbursts.

"Can I hear it again? Ernie? Can I hear it again?"

Validated, encouraged, again told the pause had ended by words spoken by Paul, Frank engaged, touched the screen, watched, listened and smiled. *You da man Ernie.*

"Do you have a copy of Seals and Croft from '76, when you called them out for their religious beliefs, with you? I'd love to hear that one again."

Enthused, Frank answered, quickly, loudly. "No. Not with me. I can get it and come back. Want me to? I will. No problem. It's a classic. My second favorite. I'm happy to go home, retrieve it and come back. Want me to?"

Paul smiled. His friend was deluded, but happy and who was Paul to judge?

Seals and Croft was his second favorite, second only to Dean Martin. Dean was Paul's favorite as well. A classic. Not planned, an accident, a classic.

When Frank was learning his craft, he traveled to Las Vegas and bought tickets to see Dean Martin, the happy, crooning, drunk. In the spirit of the show, Frank drank six Manhattans, and by the time, Dean took the stage, they were both drunk. In between songs, while he sipped his copper-colored drink, Dean attempted to entertain the audience with jokes, jokes that were old fashioned, and to the sober, not very funny. Frank was old school and not sober, so the jokes told by the drunk on-stage were extremely funny to the drunk in the audience. Dean told a joke, the audience, save one member, sat in silence, while Frank roared with laughter.

Years after he laughed at Dean, Frank bought a long-playing Dean Martin record album titled *An Evening of Music, Laughter and Hard Liquor (Live at the Sands Hotel)*. As he listened, the music sounded fuzzily familiar and when Dean told a joke between the second and third songs, he heard the beautiful music of his own laughter. Seven times in eight minutes, Frank's laughter punctuated the silence and sounded a solo clearer than any of Frank's other recordings. It was so evident and Frank's laugh so distinct, when Paul first heard the recording, he immediately knew his friend was in Las Vegas and on the recording. Frank called it a duet. *Dean and Frank. No, not Frank Sinatra. Dean and me.* He called the recording label and asked that his name be included in the album jacket in the event the recording was re-issued and after hearing chuckles nearly as loud as the laughs Frank contributed to Dean's record, was told, "No."

"No Frank, don't go home and get it now." I smiled. Sincerely. "Seals and Croft. I remember it. I can close my eyes and hear you. *Baha'i? What's that? Play Summer Breeze please.* Next time bring it with you. It's a classic."

"Yeah it's one of my favorites. That and *Tonya, you're America's queen,* at the 94 Ice Championships. I'll bring that one too. Any other requests?"

"Nope. You choose."

Frank looked puzzled. "I lose?"

More loudly. "No, you choose."

"Thanks, I heard that better. I don't hear so well."

"Really?"

"Huh?"

"Whatever you choose is fine, Frank."

"Okay. I'll stop by tomorrow with my favorites. Maybe I'll bring my portable turntable so we can listen to my duet with Deano. You'll still be here, tomorrow won't you?"

"I think so Frank. I hope so. If I'm required to live one more day to hear your favorites collection, that's what I'll need to do."

Frank was compiling a mental list of his favorites when he reached the door. He turned to look at his old friend and assure him that he'd deliver the goods and bring the best of Frank, and for the first time, saw that Paul was dying, really dying. He was gray, mottled, his cheeks sunken, his hair recently thin and wispy and his eyes glossy, without focus. His hands were gaunt and shook under the sheets, creating small waves of white. Not knowing if his lifelong pal would live to hear Frank's favorites, Frank smiled, listened for a strong heartbeat, optimism or hope, but his hearing was impaired and he heard nothing. "Thanks for pushing the Plymouth, Paul."

"Not a problem, Frank. Glad I could help."

Frank inserted index fingers into his ears and removed them quickly, clearing his listening passages. He didn't understand the question, but answered as best he could. "I think she's 12, but I don't know."

Knowing words wouldn't be heard or understood, Paul offered a thumbs-up. As he watched Frank disappear down the hall, Paul smiled, mumbled *You da man*, and waited for his next guest.

Belle rushed into the room, checked bags, those that accepted what was discharged and those that supplied nourishment and relief from pain and asked, "You okay?"

"I'm fine for a guy who's got hours and days, not months and years."

"That's all any of us has."

"Trade?"

"Trades aren't permitted. Sorry. I'll simply give you what I've got while I'm here."

"Thanks, Belle. I appreciate it."

Belle adjusted the blankets that covered Paul's disappearing body, making sure his long narrow feet did not escape their warmth. She looked around the room, satisfied she had done what could be done, put her hands on her hips and asked a question without words. Paul answered.

"Will I know when it's close?"

"I don't know Paul. I've never died. It's the great mystery. Until you're there you don't know, and after you've been, you can't tell those who remain."

"I'll try."

"What I can tell you is, my patients who have died, have done so peacefully. No thrashing, no screaming. They peacefully passed on. They took in one breath, two breaths, millions of breaths, and then, take no more. Chests which lifted and expanded for generations, are still. Many die with a smile on their face. If they were smiling, it couldn't have been bad. You think?"

"If I'm not smiling, lift the corners of my mouth please. Let me send a positive message, even after I've gone. Maybe Mary won't worry about me or be concerned about what happens to her after she takes her last breath."

Belle squeezed a covered foot, but Paul was looking the other way and had no feeling in his feet, so didn't appreciate the gesture. Practicing for death, he smiled. "Would you send in Mary?"

Mary walked into the room carrying her ever present iPad. She wore golf shorts, sandals and a collared, white tee-shirt. Her tan, compromised by visits to the hospital and her husband's bedroom which served as a hospice, was fading. Even so, it was apparent that she was an active, healthy, 74 year old who enjoyed fresh air and the sun. She set her iPad on the table and asked, "What do you want me to say today on your Caring Bridge site?"

When Paul was diagnosed and told time was short, that he'd likely celebrated his last Christmas and birthday, he and Mary told the kids and a few close friends about the diagnosis, but tired of answering the phone and kind people with questions. They wanted to know and Paul and Mary wanted them to know, they were just too tired, physically and emotionally, to answer the same questions, hour after hour, day after day, week after week, so, Mary created a Caring Bridge page for Paul.

Caring Bridge is an internet site dedicated to communications between the sick and those who are concerned about the sick. The afflicted if able, or those close to the afflicted, post information on the internet and those who are concerned or simply curious, are able to access the posted information. A Caring Bridge site is mutable, updated as diagnoses change, surgeries are performed or recoveries occur.

After Mary and Paul tired of answering telephone calls, Mary created Paul's page and on that page, she wrote:

Paul has been diagnosed with lung cancer. It is Stage IV. The cancer has spread beyond his lungs and the prognosis is not good. But, he has not given up. He has wonderful doctors and they are charting a treatment course that will be, like the cancer, aggressive, but unlike the cancer, infused with hope. Paul is hospitalized at Mercy Hospital. We don't know how long he will remain in the hospital, because at this time, we don't know how he will respond to the treatment. The doctors expect he will be released within a week, but expectations are simply that, expectations. We very much appreciate your concern, warm wishes and heart-felt prayers. We will update this site whenever there is new information and will continue to do so until Paul is back on the golf course.

Two years later, Mary looked at Paul's Caring Bridge page and read that she had posted updates 522 times. When Paul was in the hospital, there was nothing more to say, the lines remained blurred, the prognosis continued guarded, so Mary updated Paul's page infrequently. When she returned home with Paul after a lung lobe had been removed, her telephone had 42 messages and her email account had 31 unread messages that inquired about Paul's health, Mary updated the Caring Bridge site and for a glorious day, they received no telephone calls or email messages asking *What's new?* Four days after she updated the page, she received 12 telephone calls and received 14 email messages. On that fourth day, she posted new information on Caring Bridge and her phone and computer were silent for the following two days. A quick learner, Mary learned a lesson. Post daily and avoid telephone calls and emails. So, she posted daily.

The posts reflected the mood that consumed Mary when she wrote. Some posts were brief, hurried. *No change. Paul is still home, still going to the doctor daily, but no change.* Some were upbeat. *Paul had a great day today. No pain, no coughing jags, no need to worry.* Some were depressing. *Paul is sleeping. It seems as though he sleeps all the time, unless he's coughing, writhing in pain or telling me what to do. Keep him in your prayers.* Some were hopeful. *Paul seems to be getting stronger. The treatments seem to be helping. We went out for dinner and I almost forgot he was sick.* Some were not. *It never ends. A doctor's visit, followed by a lab appointment, followed by another doctor's appointment, followed by a trip to the pharmacy. Although we remain hopeful, it's hard. Maybe tomorrow will be a better day. I doubt it, but hope so.*

Mary lifted her iPad and held it before her husband who was imprisoned by side-rails and disease. "Caring Bridge. What do you want me to say today?"

"Tell them I died and after three months of seclusion, you'll arrange for a winter funeral. That'll keep 'em from bothering you, and you won't need to post every day."

"Are you kidding me? If I posted that, I'd be swamped with casseroles, sympathy calls and grandkids prematurely grieving Pop's passing."

"Then just tell them to *Fuck off.*"

Mary's smile disappeared and a blush appeared on her neck, making its way from her collar to her chin. "Why would you say such a thing? They're just concerned."

"I just want to die in peace. No responsibilities, no duties. I want to be left alone." Paul closed his eyes, turned his face from Mary and felt a tear fall from his left eye and travel down his cheek to the bed. After he tried to erase the track of his tear with the sleeve of his pajama top, he looked at Mary and unsuccessfully tried to smile.

"Are you okay?"

Paul took some time to formulate his answer. He thought he knew why he said what he had said, but wanted to make certain, before he told Mary. And if he was right, he wanted to find the right words, words that wouldn't evoke fear or sympathy.

"Just now, I realized, I'm going to die. Not in the next decade, not next year, but soon. The doctors told me that long ago and I've admitted in conversations with others and myself, that the time remaining was short, but they were just words. I heard it, I said it, but down deep, in my heart of hearts, I didn't believe it. And three minutes ago, it became real. Something Belle said triggered it. She said something and I said to myself, *This is real, you're going to die. Not someone else, not a character on T.V., you, which is me.* It's scary. And sad."

Before Mary could formulate a response and attempt to comfort the terminally uncomfortable, Alyson walked into the room. Her shoulders were rounded, her head tipped to her chest. Her eyes darted from her mom to her dad and then to the floor. Her hands were balled into fists and her jaw set and tight. She cleared her throat and with a voice that cracked as she spoke, delivered bad news. "Frank's dead. Left here, got in his car across the street and died behind the wheel, with his keys in his hands."

You da man, Ernie.

chapter fifteen

After the shock disappeared, Paul jokingly suggested they delay transportation of Frank's corpse to the funeral home until later, so they could share a coffin, funeral service and cemetery plot, but when he envisioned an eternity of *You da man*, he changed his advice and suggested the body be delivered to the undertaker *post haste*.

After Frank's body was removed from his car and his car removed from the front of Paul's prison, Mary answered the question Paul had asked an hour and a half earlier. "You know you're going to die; so do I. Frank didn't and he's dead. It's all a question of timing and preparation. You're better prepared for *whenever* the time arrives."

Paul had forgotten the question he earlier asked Mary. His fear had abated. Frank's death diverted his attention from his impending death to Frank's consummated death, from speculation to confirmation. He was a good friend, a lifelong friend, a friend who had made him smile minutes before he took his final breath, a good friend. Paul was saddened by Frank's death, shocked by its suddenness and surprised that it happened without a sign, a map, a predictor. Frank left Paul's room with a smile and a purpose, made a commitment to return and then died. No warning. No hint. No hysterical, emotional goodbye. On his feet one moment, and the next, on his back in the crematorium's oven. *Boom. Gone. Quick. Ashes.*

"He was going to bring me a compilation of his favorite recorded outbursts tomorrow. I guess he won't be doing that tomorrow. At least not here. Maybe he'll have it waiting for me on the other side. I'll open my eyes and he'll be standing there with his iPad in the ready position, like he did two hours ago. I won't know if I'm dead or reliving today. Spooky." Paul laughed, his laugh became a cough and his cough, then a jag.

When the gagging ended, the pain subsided and Paul regained his breath, he said, "And if Frank's there, and it's an eternity of *You da man*, am I in Heaven or Hell?"

Paul was making light of Frank's death and silently asked himself *Why?* He was a sad sack, but a nice guy, a lifelong friend. He just died, unexpectedly, in front of Paul's home, minutes after he left Paul's bedside, attempting to provide Paul comfort, and yet, Paul laughed? *Why?* The answer was kinda simple.

Frank left no family to mourn his passing. No surviving children or grandkids would grieve at his coffin or sob at his funeral. There was no surviving spouse to roll over and wake in bed, alone for the first time in decades. She wouldn't reach for her husband, miss the warm spot on his side of the bed or cry tears of loneliness, because she didn't exist, Frank hadn't married. Dash Crofts, who Frank had asked about *Bai Hai*, and Ernie Els wouldn't notice and few would recognize the name, if Frank's obituary was published in the local paper. Frank was kind, but he had a limited following, no emotional investments and few would cry.

Frank's death wouldn't affect what remained of Paul's life to any appreciable degree. Paul didn't have much left to be affected. Frank would no longer wait in line to see Paul, wouldn't play recordings of his voice shouted over the hysteria of the masses, but someone else would take his place in line and another would entertain Paul with recollections from concerts or games, and likely those recollections will be more interesting than *You da man, Ernie*. Paul liked Frank, but with only days remaining, his absence wouldn't matter significantly.

Paul had attended graveyard services. He stood near the box that held his father, mother and close friends, 15 feet from a mound of dirt covered by green carpet, and listened to a minister or priest read Bible verses and command the body to the earth and the soul to Heaven. When he dropped a flower on the box and walked away, he looked over his shoulder and saw that the box and its contents, his mom, dad or friend remained, alone, that they hadn't left with the mourners. As he drove toward home over the narrow tar roads that dissected the cemetery, he looked in the mirror and saw the men with shovels scoop dirt and bury the dead and knew the darkness in the box, was getting darker, but it didn't matter their eyes were closed, their brains dead. At home, after the service, when darkness enveloped his home and bitter cold turned dirt into frozen, brown concrete, when people crawled between sheets and animals huddled together for warmth, when the only movement in the cemetery was from wind-blown leaves or scraps of paper, he pictured the mound of dirt on top of the box and the lifeless body inside, alone. He had always been fascinated by life's continuation, while something once living, no longer participated. *Here today, gone tomorrow.* He drove to work, his dad remained motionless, underground, in a box. He laughed at Bill Murray on the screen, his mom remained motionless, underground, in a box. The doctors told him he had cancer and his parents remained motionless, underground, in a box.

Death's novelty died. It was old, familiar. Soon, Frank would join Paul's mother, his father and deceased friends, motionless, underground, in a box, but Paul wasn't moved by Frank's isolation, his inability to move or shout over the crowd, because he had simply done what Paul would do soon. *I'm coming, my friend.*

Frank's death, unfortunate and unforeseen, wasn't devastating to Paul or anyone else. The light went off and couldn't be relit, but the sun still rose and all those who remained, could still see.

"Sleep in peace, my friend. See you soon. *You da man.*"

Paul saw that Mary continued to hold her iPad, which was still open to Paul's Caring Bridge page. Resigned to death and peacefully invited by a friend, temporarily unafraid, Paul smiled. "Tell them I'm dying, but awake and smiling, pain-free and mourning the passing of a good man and great friend. Tell them he left too soon and taught us all to cherish life, because it can end abruptly, without notice. Tell them I loved my lifelong friend and close with, *You da man, Ernie* No explanation, just, *You da man, Ernie.*"

As Mary punched keys, Paul closed his eyes and with eyes wide shut, saw two teenaged boys in a 1941 Plymouth. The windows were open, the boys' hair tussled by wind, their smiles wide. They laughed. With innocence electrified by youth and compromised by experience, they traveled through time on their way to tomorrow.

Paul slept and woke an hour after he closed his eyes. Belle sat in the chair next to Paul's bed. She was watching a muted television which provided dialogue in subtitles that appeared on the screen. When Paul cleared his throat, Belle looked away from the television and to Paul and welcomed him back with a smile.

"So, I'm not dead?"

"Nope. Like me, you're alive and kicking."

"Unlike Frank. Anyone know what happened to him?"

Belle wiped Paul's mouth clean, combed his hair with long, thin fingers and answered. "I talked to a cop who stopped by, after Alyson called and Frank had been taken from his car. He said it was probably a heart attack. Nothing suspicious. At his age, they suspect his heart stopped and he died quietly."

"I wonder if they'll try to confirm the cause of death."

"Why? What difference does it make? He didn't leave anyone behind and there were no suspicious signs. Autopsies are expensive and performed only when a loved one asks or there are suspicious circumstances surrounding the death. My guess is he's already ashes."

"I wonder if there will be a service?"

"Don't know. Did he have anyone who would make arrangements?"

Not Ernie, not Dash, not Paul. "Nope. People said *Hi*, but he was pretty much alone, with his recordings."

"Sad."

"Yup."

Paul pitied his dead friend. When alive, Frank was effervescent, yet shallow, loud, yet voiceless. He was happy, but had little to say and no one listened when he did. But, because he always smiled, always found joy in his next pursuit, Paul never felt sorry for him. In spite of all that Paul had and all that Frank did not have, Frank was the happier of the two. His life was simple and sprinkled with glee.

Frank's death highlighted his relative isolation and insignificance. He was alone. No one would stand in the cemetery while he was lowered in a hole; no one would hear dirt scatter when it landed on an oak box encased in a concrete tomb. He was alone.

"Belle, please ask Mary to step in." Paul smiled. It was if he was at his office and Belle his secretary. *Belle, please ask Mary to step in.*

Belle walked out and Mary walked in. She stood before Paul, smiled and awaited instructions.

"Would you please find out if Frank left any instructions. If he didn't, tell the funeral home that he'll be a part of my service. Our service. If they cremate him, timing will be unimportant. If I last a week, that's fine, if I last a year, that's fine. When people pray for my soul, they can pray for Frank's. I'll write something about Frank and it can be read at the service. He lived alone, he shouldn't be sent off to the hereafter alone."

Paul had a goal, a purpose other than waiting to die. He felt alive and for a moment thought he felt his feet. *Nah.* "Can you get me paper and a pen?"

Mary left the room while Paul took mental notes for a eulogy to be spoken at his funeral. *Yup. Yeah. That's good.*

Five minutes after her exit, Mary re-entered. "Thurston's says Frank's body is in its basement. He'll be in cold storage until they determine if he left instructions or if instructions will be given by next-of-kin. If there are no instructions, he'll be cremated and buried in a nameless plot at Calvary Cemetery. According to the guy I talked to, a court order could resolve things as you want, and it could be obtained easily, so long as there aren't heirs."

Paul asked Mary to call Tom Pertler, the disbarred lawyer, who knew how to speak *legalize,* even if he couldn't practice law, and ask him to find out what needed to be done to obtain a court order authorizing Paul to take possession of Frank's ashes and send him to the other world in a joint church service. He gave Mary the name of two sympathetic, common-sense judges and suggested Tom call one and ask, on Paul's behalf, what could be done. He asked her to give him the paper and pen she held and watched her leave the room to do as requested. Paul put pen to paper and wrote:

Frank Nistler. I had the good fortune of being born near and raised with Frank Nistler. And I have the good fortune of dying with him and catching the same bus to the hereafter with him. We lived and died together. Like Butch and Sundance or Bonnie and Clyde.

Frank was born in 1939 and died in 2015. He served his country in the United States' Army. He never married, never sired children. He always smiled.

Many of you didn't know Frank. He was always here, but you likely didn't see him. He wanted it that way. He was unassuming and mostly quiet, except when he performed. You might not know what Frank looked like, but you probably know what he sounded like.

He performed with all of the greats. Seals and Croft. Elvis. Arnold Palmer. The Wild, the Gophers, the Twins and Timberwolves. They performed better when Frank was there, and he let them and us know how much he appreciated their performances. Without Frank, Seals and Croft were just music, Arnold Palmer, just golf and the Twins, Wolves, Gophers and Wild, just sports teams. With Frank, they were all more than they were without him. He was the exclamation point, the epilogue, the 10th inning of a nine-inning game, the fourth period of a hockey game, the fifth quarter of a basketball game, the coda, the encore.

Frank Nistler was my friend and he had the temerity to time his death so that I wouldn't be alone, here or hereafter. Thank you, Frank, for now, for yesterday and for tomorrow. **You da man.**

chapter sixteen

As Paul set the pen and paper down on the bed next to him, Mary told him she had called Tom and he had agreed to do as asked.

"And I hope he knows time is of the essence."

"He was here yesterday, Paul. He knows."

"Yeah, you're right. He'll do it fast."

Mary reached for the pen and paper that rested on the slope of the mattress that led to Paul, a slope which became less pronounced every day, as Paul wasted away and the depression his shrinking body created became shallower. Before Mary's extended hand reached the paper, Paul reached for it, grabbed it and said, "You can read it when I'm dead. And, leave the paper and pen here. I may have more to say."

"Ouch. A little sensitive about potential criticism? I'll be kind."

Paul responded sheepishly. He'd been too quick, too insensitive. "I'm sorry. Didn't mean to be so short, even though I don't have the time to be anything but. Life is more fun with surprises and maybe death can be less horrific if there are some surprises. If I write something and you don't read it until I'm gone, it's almost like I'll be talking from the grave. Fun. Surprising. And trust me, at this stage, editorial comments wouldn't phase me. I think I'm past that."

Mary grinned. "Watch what you write. Remember, by the time we read it, you can't take it back or offer another interpretation."

"I'll be careful. Must be. It'll be my legacy."

"No, it won't. Your legacy is your family, the people you've touched with kindness and the insightful, sweet words you've already spoken. That's what people will remember long after you're gone."

"Maybe that's the punch line to a long life. Perhaps 20 years from now, people will remember what you think they'll remember, my lifetime of kind words and good deeds, but at the end of conversations spoken in the weeks after my last breath, they'll say, *And, can you believe what he wrote while lying in bed waiting to die?*"

Before Mary responded, Paul thought about what he had said, and smiled. It was almost over, but he had time to change his life and how people remembered him. 75 years. Not much time. Too little time, but if he was remembered long after he died, his impact could be stretched from 75 years to 300 years. If he impacted people 225 years after he died, 75% of his impact had yet to be experienced. *It's not nearly over. It's early. I'm just starting.*

Mary waited while Paul pondered. When he turned his face from Mary to the window, it was apparent he was thinking, formulating, reflecting. After finishing his thoughts, Paul turned from the window to Mary. He said nothing, but his gaze made suggestions. *Ready? Please speak.* And Mary answered. "Well, you write and I'll wait like everyone else, to hear what you have to say."

And he wrote.

Please, don't misunderstand me. I love life. It's been a wonderful life, but I'm fascinated by death, in particular, my death. It's the riddle that can't be answered by anyone who might read my ramblings. By the time you read this, I'll know the answer; you won't. You're alive, I'm not. I'm dead. Sorry.

But, as I lay on my hospice bed with my body failing and my mind temporarily sharp, I'm fascinated by what I may discover in hours, days or weeks. I'm too much of an optimist, a believer in good, to be afraid. Either there's nothing or there's something, and if there's something, it's constructed, managed and maintained by God, and I believe God is good. Goodness is forgiveness and happiness, not punitive and despair. God is good and in control, so, I'm optimistic.

I feel like a 12-year old boy in front of a tent, under the stars, with my best friend. We'd discuss infinity and where it all began. We'd look at the ceiling dotted with dots of light and ask where it ended, and if it ended, what was on the other side. We wondered how it all began, how it was created and what happened before it happened. We had no answers, except to say, We probably won't know until we're dead.

And the wait is nearly over. My energy diminishes while my excitement grows. In days, I may be able to walk on the stars and tap on the wall that is the end. I may meet the Creator and see how it began and what was, before there was anything. Voyageur found Neptune years after it left Earth; I may find the end of the universe in days. It's fascinating. I'm excited about the ride, the answers.

Paul considered reading and editing his message, but decided against it. *Not enough time. As is.* And it was probably good enough. Lawyer training. He'd written hundreds of legal briefs and thousands of letters as a lawyer. The words he chose when he wrote letters, affidavits and legal arguments, the words he spoke in the courtroom, determined how a case was resolved, so he chose carefully. Editing, unnecessary.

Ladies and gentlemen, evil still lurks. It's out there and it's my hope that the investigators who wrongfully concluded Ron Scott was evil, hear the music, recognize Mr. Scott's innocence and find the person responsible for the death of two children. The words were chosen carefully and Ron was free.

I'm sorry. I know you loved your Mother and did what you could do. The words were spoken carefully and he was married. For 48 years.

It's just a game, a game you play well. Have fun and leave the court with your game intact, quick and hard, win or lose. The words were spoken and Lauren prevailed 2-6, 7-5, 6-0.

It was his nature and his training. He was careful. *No need to edit. As is.*

Paul set the paper artistically soiled with ink on the bed, on the side nearer the window, away from clutching hands and greedy eyes. When he turned from the paper to the door, he saw Mary standing sentry, acting as gatekeeper. "Alice is here."

Paul combed his hair with his fingers, cleaned the corners of his mouth with a thumb and index-finger, cleared his throat, attempted to blink tired from tired eyes, pinched color into his cheeks and laughed so imperceptibly, only he heard it. "Send her in." He laughed. "And shut the door." Before Mary walked away, Paul added, "And Mary, I love you."

Mary turned for the kitchen and then back towards Paul, grinned and said, "I know. Too late to be jealous now."

When Alice walked into the room, smiling, sparkling, nearly dancing, Paul's heart stopped. So pretty, so lively, so fresh. *Beat heart. Beat.*

Alice was evidence that first loves never die. Paul's first love never died and he suspected when he took his last breath, it would leave with him. It wouldn't die. Thankfully, it had found its proper place.

They met in seventh grade. Band. She played flute, Paul banged drums. They were friendly, not friends, until ninth grade, when a fellow-flutist began dating a fellow-drummer. Their social circles intersected and they were each members of a group of 12 that did things together. Convenient friendship morphed into close friends when the flutist who dated the drummer died. Before her death, the fellow flutist was a closet worrier, a depressed and frightened girl and when the adolescent drummer said, *It's been nice*, her depression sprang into dark action and she cut her wrists and died.

Alice was devastated. She took the death of her friend and fellow flutist hard. Paul suspected Alice suspected she was depressed as well. She mourned for her friend and feared for herself. Paul went to the funeral and sat in the pew, next to Alice. When she cried, Paul comforted her with an arm around her shoulder and a tissue. When sniffles became sobs, Paul massaged Alice's shoulder and whispered, *It'll be all right*, over and over, until because of or in spite of Paul's comfort, she stopped crying.

Paul began to pick Alice out in the crowd. As he banged sticks against a drum skin, he watched her manipulate her flute. He counted the number of seconds between breaths as she played, and noticed that although other girls rested their flutes on their laps between notes played and notes to-be-played, Alice kept her flute high, inches below her wonderful mouth. When she had a cold and wiped a red nose, Paul knew, he could see from the other side of the band room. He knew she wore eight different sweaters, three pair of shoes, four skirts and mixed and matched the outfits, so she could wear a different combination for 96 consecutive days. In tenth grade, Alice rolled her ankle and walked with a wrap and a limp. Paul offered to carry her books to and from class, and Alice said, "Yes, Paul, you're such a good friend."

During the first quarter of eleventh grade, Paul dated Mary Fifer, who was blonde like Alice, but much taller than Alice. It didn't work. During the second quarter, he dated Lynn Jones, who played the flute and was the same height as Alice, but she rested her flute on her lap between notes. It didn't work. In the spring of 1956, just a few months before he was to complete his junior year of high school, Paul bought a flower, rented a tuxedo and brought Lisa Long to prom, but when he arrived, Alice said *Hello*, and Paul forgot that he had brought Lisa to the dance.

Alice dated the same boy in eleventh and twelfth grade. He was a year older and a prick. Paul didn't understand Alice's fascination. He had dirt under his fingernails, wore soiled pants, spoke with an edge in his voice, wasn't friendly or all that nice looking and waited impatiently for Alice after football games when the band played, looking and acting as if he was drunk. He was a prick.

On October 14, 1956, at 8:55 p.m., Alice found Paul at a concession stand near the end zone of Goodrich Field, where the Tornadoes played football and the band played halftime. Her right cheek was red and she was crying. She asked Paul if he would drive her home and he did.

They didn't drive directly to Alice's home. They drove around. And around. And around.

Tony, Alice's boyfriend had asked her to leave the game before it was over, and when she said she couldn't, he hit her in the face, with a closed fist. It wasn't the first time.

During the following 90-days, Paul drove Alice to school, drove her home, and when he was through with work, picked her up at home and took her to eat. He sang to her, counseled her, cared for her. While he gave Alice the strength she needed to fly without regret or pain, Paul fell in love. He may have always loved her, the way she held her flute, the breaths she took between bars, her smile, her face, her hair, her voice, her sweetness and resilience, but when she left his car 60 days after she was slugged in the face, he knew. *Damn it, I love her.*

Paul didn't try to kiss Alice, didn't ask her to dance or tell her he was in love, with her. He knew she needed time and relied on his friendship and he didn't want it compromised by affection that ultimately led to the bedroom. He waited, satisfied that he was close to her.

Paul's grandmother lived in Texas during the winter, and during Christmas break in 1956, Paul and his family drove to Texas to escape the cold, snow and Anoka. Paul didn't want to go, to leave Alice and asked to stay home alone, but was told *No.*

When Paul's family returned to -26 degrees and Paul jump-started his car, as it warmed, he called Alice to tell her he was home and wanted to see her. She was upbeat, happy. When Paul asked if she wanted to get a bite to eat, Alice broke his heart. "Sorry, I can't. I have a date with Tom Schiff. We dated last week and I think I really like him. Sorry."

Paul knew the apology was not for breaking his heart. She didn't know; she had no idea.

Paul started his third year of college, when Alice and Tom married.

Paul started law school a week after Alice gave birth to her first child.

Paul stepped off a helicopter in South Vietnam two days after Alice delivered her fourth child and she and Tom celebrated their sixth anniversary.

Paul didn't talk to Alice after he was told *I really like him* for nearly 50 years.

When Paul was 28, soon after he proposed to Mary, nearly 11 years after Alice announced her new relationship and broke Paul's heart, Paul slowed his truck as he crossed railroad tracks and looked to his left and saw Alice, behind the wheel traveling in the opposite direction. His heart stopped.

On September 11, 1991, Paul traveled to Zion Lutheran Church, to donate blood. As his nurse swabbed his arm with cotton and alcohol, he looked toward the door and saw Alice in a nurse's uniform, tending to another donor. His heart stopped.

At their fiftieth reunion, Paul arrived early with Cliff and a half-century after his heart was broken, worried Alice would attend and crush him again. Paul watched the front door and when Alice walked in, his heart stopped and he asked Cliff to find a ride home with someone else, so that he could leave.

Paul was ashamed of his unrequited love in his teens, twenties and thirties, but when he turned 40, he told Mary, Cliff and anyone else willing to listen. He didn't long for Alice, wouldn't leave Mary for Alice, had no interest in resurrection, but felt compelled to tell the story that was an important chapter in his life. At a Bar Association dinner in 2000, Paul met a lawyer who had recently married Alice's sister. When Paul was introduced to the lawyer's wife, Alice's sister, proud and uninhibited, set free by age, he smiled broadly and said, *I was in love with your sister.*

When she responded with *I know*, Paul knew that everyone, including Alice, knew.

Alice's husband, Tom Schiff died in 2013. Paul struggled with his response and ultimately decided, he had been there before and he should be there then. When he walked into the church and saw Alice with her grown children, his heart stopped. She saw him and smiled.

Tom's death had been years in the making, he had been ravaged by a slow moving, incurable cancer that took his voice and mind, so his death was more liberating than devastating. Paul sat in the back of the church and listened to Tom's children and the pastor eulogize him. Paul tried, but couldn't hear, couldn't internalize the kind words, couldn't forgive Tom. He didn't hate Tom, he understood him, recognized his attraction and resented him for what Paul believed he had taken from him. When the pastor asked the congregation to pray for Tom's soul, Paul folded his hands and joined in the prayer. It was over. Tom married Alice. He won. Paul was alive; Tom was dead. Paul won.

As Alice and her family filed out of the church, she again caught Paul's eye and smiled. Paul, healed by a smile, Alice's ghost exorcised by a smile, smiled.

As Paul was about to step from the narthex into the cold, he felt a hand on his shoulder. He turned, his heart stopped and he was 17. Alice smiled at Paul for the third time in half-an-hour and said, "Boy, you work fast."

Paul returned Alice's warm smile, took her hand in his and said, "Alice, this is my wife, Mary."

They renewed their friendship. Paul accepted that friendship is all they ever had and would be all they would ever have. They had meals together, took long drives together, talked about their past and future. Mary was always with, always participated, always understood.

But, every time Paul saw her, his heart stopped.

Beat heart. Beat.

"Hello Alice."

"Gosh. In bed, in hospice, no sun, no fresh air, and still the most handsome man in Anoka." She smiled and blushed on cue. It was a talent. In high school, over a pizza, someone would ask her to blush, and she could and would. On cue. A real talent.

She wore a wide brimmed hat, had during the day, for thirty years. Her skin was fair and the sun burned her and blemished her with a cancerous lesion when she was 42. She had it removed and every day thereafter, ventured outside during the summer months, while the sun was high, only after applying sunscreen to her exposed skin and a wide brimmed hat to her pretty head.

When his heart started beating and then went from too fast to slow, Paul said something he had wanted to say for almost 60 years, but hadn't had the courage. With death peaking around the corner and so little to lose, he figured it was time. "Do you know, that when we were in high school, I was madly in love with you?"

"Yes, I do. Cliff told me before I married Tom. Just in case. My sister told me. Janice Sjoberg told me. Others told me on an almost weekly basis over the last 60 years."

"Well, I thought it was time I told you."

"Paul, you told me many times. Every time I saw you, you made it clear. You couldn't look at me, and when you accidently saw me, your knees buckled and upper lip quivered. It was clear. Sorry."

Paul couldn't blush on cue, but he could still blush, and he did. "When did you first know?"

"After I started dating Tom. You and I did so much together and I thought we would continue to do things together. When you avoided me and left conversations every time I joined them, I knew."

"Sorry. It was childish."

"No, it was sweet."

Old, crusty, dying, Paul barely remembered sweet. He said nothing, waiting for Alice to finish.

"Tom and I had a wonderful life together. We raised four great kids and I loved him until he died. But, I never knew you cared for me in ways other than the ways friends care for one another, until it was too late. You never told me, never let me know. By the time I knew, I was in love with Tom. It was too late."

"Always late. The story of my life."

"Not true. You did everything that was supposed to be done, when it was to be done. You went to college, law school and served our country in war. You married Mary, raised three wonderful children and lived a good life. You weren't late for me, you were right on time for the others."

"You were always perceptive and so often right. How'd we drift apart for 55 years?"

"We had other things to do. We didn't have time for each other. You found the time when I needed you and I'm here now when you're in need."

"Mary was a good wife; is a good wife. I love her and am glad we met, married and stayed together almost 50 years. I have no regrets. None. But I certainly understand why I fell in love with you. Tom was a lucky man."

"And Mary a lucky woman."

They talked about friends who played in band, friends with whom they shared pizza and conversation, friends who married and divorced, friends who moved away and returned home to die. Alice remembered the songs Paul sang and Paul tried to sing one then, but his throat was unwilling, and instead he was only able to cough a note or two. Alice smiled, she understood, told him not to worry, that for almost 60 years, she had been able to close her eyes and hear him sing. "And I'll hear you sing tonight and when you are gone." She closed her eyes, moved her lips, smiled and added, "Such a beautiful voice."

Paul tired, but he fought his heavy eyelids; he didn't want Alice to leave. He knew it would be his last time. Alice knew her friend and nearly lover and sensed his need for sleep. She stood, removed her broad brimmed hat, leaned over the siderail, kissed Paul's forehead and said, "Goodbye, my friend. I love you too."

Before Alice crossed the threshold, Paul slept. His sleep was deep, his dreams vivid and romantic. They danced. They made love. He gazed into her eyes. They held hands and kissed. He told her over and over again, *I love you*. And **Mary** smiled and said, *I love you too*.

chapter
seventeen

Paul woke in the dark. *The other side? The inside of a closed box? Burned and stuffed in a bottle?* He listened for the crack of a fire, all around him or below him as he rested in an urn placed on the fireplace mantel. He listened for the sound of dirt splashing on an oak lid above him, heard nothing, pushed his hands toward the ceiling or the coffin's cotton top, discovered that he was not in a box or an urn, and turned and read the digital clock. *3:15.*

Paul found the bed's remote control and pushed the button. He sat upright at 3:16 a.m., alone. It was different, refreshing. He typically slept all night and had visitors all day. They had talked about *Eleventh Hour* care, a person at his bedside 24 hours daily, a person to be there when his heart stopped beating and his need for oxygen ended, when he moved to the other side, but decided it wasn't time, that the end wasn't *that* near, that more evidence of inevitability was needed before family sprinted towards the finish line. So, he was in his bed with siderails and no one else was near. Rarely was he awake and alone. He was and it felt good. If he had the strength, he could leave his bed and clip his toenails, and no one could tell him *No*. If he had the strength and desire, he could touch himself and relieve sexual hunger, and no one would blush with embarrassment or tell him *No*. No witnesses, no supervisors, no killjoys. It felt good.

Paul considered turning on the television to search for a sixties series, *Bonanza, Big Valley* or *Gunsmoke*, but knew if he did, the sound would stir someone, somewhere else in the house, and his independence would be compromised, and he would no longer be able to clip his toenails or touch himself, so left the television screen black and stared into the darkness. *3:17*. He lifted the bedding with his right hand and his left dipped below the covers and slid down across his ribs and belly and stopped at the waistband of his pajama bottoms. He stretched the elastic belt as his fingers reached lower in search of a friend. He found it. Soft. Small, almost non-existent. Uninterested. He turned on the television.

Dick Cavett spoke to an older, distinguished looking woman who explained that she wanted to be remembered for her love of life and the joy she spread through her music. She sang and Paul asked himself, *What's that? Who's she?* He changed the channel. Miss Barbara Stanwick, in a denim shirt, wearing a bolo-tie and dungarees, pleaded with Jarrod to intervene and protect his hot-headed brother, Nick Barkley, from himself. *Click.* Tim Allen was Santa Claus, in August, *Click,* Bernie Sanders proposed free college education and health care for all Americans and *Click*, Trump was mocking an opponent by suggesting that because his hands were small, something else was likely small. As he held his orange paws in front of the camera, he looked at his groin and said, *No problem down there for me, that I can assure you.*

Paul silenced the television with the mute button, revisited his fifth appendage, confirmed his disappointment and cleared his throat. *3:19.* With aid from the light off the television screen, he read what he wrote the day before. *Pretty good.*

He wrote. *It's amazing. Things change. Years ago, if I had awakened at 3:00 in the morning, I'd have panicked. I needed sleep. Too many important things to do, without adequate sleep, I can't do them. Panic would have raised my blood pressure and my heart rate and the chance of returning to sleep was lost. I'd toss and turn, refusing to look at the clock to determine how much sleep I'd missed and how close it was until the alarm sounded. Damn. Left side, right side, on my back, left, right. Shit. **Now**, it makes no difference. 3:17 a.m. is no different than 3:17 p.m. At 3:17 a.m., it's dark and I'm alone, but the difference is marginal. I wake when I wake and stay awake until I fall asleep. Nothing on my calendar, except a date that is moving, hopefully way out, but frighteningly, closer. Not a problem. No panic. No big deal. 3:21.*

Alice Hanson, now Alice Schiff, but I prefer to remember her from 1956, not the decades between then and now, visited me today. She kissed me. It was the first time she has ever kissed me, and although it was a kiss for comfort, a friendly smooch, a platonic peck on the forehead, it fulfilled an item on my personal bucket list. Watch the Australian Open in Melbourne, hike the foothills of Everest, donate a kidney, run a marathon, have a conversation with an ex-president, write and publish a novel, sing a duet with Paul McCartney in Liverpool, convince just one Trump supporter that he's not invincible, kiss Alice Hanson. One down, many to go.

I don't know if I would have been happy with Alice. She broke my heart when it was still developing. It never fully recovered and the broken piece forever longed-for comfort and repair from the person responsible for the breakage, Alice. I never saw Alice the way others saw her. When she appeared before me in her car, on foot or in my dreams, I saw the girl who refused to rest her flute in her lap, the girl who needed comfort when a young hooligan's drunkenness morphed into an assault, the girl who fell in love and married while I pined. I was in love with Alice, but it was the Alice of my past, the Alice of my dreams, not necessarily Alice. Is it any less real if based on history and dreams? Not for me. I always loved Alice and the love was real. I'm still 17, and still in love with Alice.

Does my love of Alice tarnish my love for Mary? No, not at all. I love my children, Alyson, Lauren and Randy, and my love for them does not diminish my love for their mother. I love Alice, but it doesn't interfere with my love for my wife. As I harbored love for Alice, I married Mary and didn't hesitate at the altar, but instead spoke my vows as quickly as they could be spoken, so I could hear the man in black with a white collar tell me as soon as possible, that Mary was my wife. When I held my children in my arms, I didn't ask God to make them like me or Alice, I prayed they would grow up to be just like their mom, Mary, kind, honest, generous, loving. When doctors told me, I was sick and would soon die, I didn't seek comfort from the woman who broke my heart and haunted me for generations, Alice, I found Mary and combatted my fears and shed tears in her arms.

I don't want Belle to wash my forehead. I want the kiss to linger and accompany me to the other side, but its importance will be diminished among the kisses, children, memories, tears and comfort that can't be washed away with a wet rag, gifts given by Mary, Alyson, Randy and Lauren.

Let's do this. Mr. DeMille, I'm ready for my close-up.

3:44. Goodnight.

Paul slept for four hours. If he dreamed, the dreams were not memorable. When he opened his eyes, he saw two televisions, two Belles, four feet tenting the bedding and two left hands reaching for his eyes. He rubbed his eyes and four became two and two became one.

"Sleep well?"

"Yes, I did. I was up in the middle of the night, but fell asleep again, without trouble."

"Me too."

Paul knew little about Belle. She stayed at Paul's home and would remain there until Paul was removed on a gurney with his face covered by a sheet. She saved his short life by removing an obstruction in his throat and washed his face, chest, back, legs, feet and…. She made camp in Alyson's former bedroom and slept when Paul slept or when the line of well-wishers was long enough to assume Paul would be accompanied by friends who could wake and alert Belle in the event of an emergency. She was reliable, kind, skilled and pleasant, always greeting Paul with a smile and leaving him with another. But, he knew little about her.

"Do you have family Belle?"

"A husband and three grown children, two grandkids and a Golden Retriever."

"Do you miss them when you're away, when you're here?"

"A bit. But my kids and husband have been here in the last couple of days. They bring me a meal and news and we catch up. So, although I'm not at home, we're in contact. It's not so bad. And it gives me the opportunity to be here, with you."

"I'm glad you're here."

"Me too."

Belle left the room and returned with a washcloth in hand. She wiped Paul's mouth clean and lifted the wet, warm cloth towards his forehead. Paul blocked Belle and the washcloth and said, "Not the forehead, at least not today."

"There's a bit of red on your forehead. Don't you want me to clean it off?"

"Nope. That's exactly what I don't want washed away." Paul smiled.

Belle smiled, returned the washcloth to the bedroom bathroom and returned to stand at the end of the bed. "Anything else I can do?"

"No, except next time your husband is here, bring him in. I'd like to tell him how lucky he is."

"Will do. Are you ready for visitors?"

"That's what I'm here for."

"I'll tell Mary and ask her to step in, so you two can figure out who gets in next."

Mary walked into the room with her iPad under her left arm. She stood next to Paul, looked at him and smiled. "I wasn't wearing lipstick yesterday."

Paul said nothing in response to the comment, because he didn't know what to say, or believed silence was more articulate than words. He asked, "Who's here?"

"The usual cast. Cliff, Randy, Alyson, Lauren, Sandy James. No Alice and Frank's still dead, so he's not here either. And a guy named Phil Scott is here. He said you guys were in the service together."

Phil and Paul served in Vietnam together. Phil was Paul's little brother in the jungle. He enlisted after graduating from high school, and because Paul did not join the effort until after law school, when they met, Paul was 26 and Phil 19. Paul's mother gave birth to a still-born child in 1947, a boy who was buried at Calvary Cemetery, without a name. When Paul met Phil, also from Anoka, also born in 1947, brown eyed, left-handed, with blonde hair, Paul considered the odds, and protected him as he would have protected his little brother, had he lived.

On patrol in 1965, likely north of the line between North and South Vietnam, Phil led the squadron through heavy jungle on a narrow trail, when Paul saw something reflect the sun and told him to stop. When Paul walked in front of Phil and located the metallic object that reflected the sun's rays, he discovered a trip-wire buried in brush that crossed the path. He clipped the wire, retreated to the bowels of the squadron and told Phil to proceed.

When the patrol unit returned to their camp that evening, Phil found Paul and thanked him. "Lieutenant, you save my life today. If you hadn't seen that wire, I'd have walked into it and set off a boobytrap that would have killed me and maybe more. I'd be dead right now, if it hadn't been for you. I owe you my life."

Paul knew Phil was right, but didn't believe in drama, especially in the jungle. "Corporal, you'd have seen the wire if I hadn't. I didn't save your life, just saved you the trouble of cutting the wire."

"I don't think so. I'd be dead had you not seen the wire."

"One, I believe you'd have seen it and would have saved your own life, had I given you the opportunity to do so, and if not, I just did my job and am not entitled to praise. We're a unit. We all have a job to do. I did mine and may have helped avert danger, but you do your job in the jungle, day-after-day, and what you do protects me and everyone else in this squad from the enemy. So, while you're thanking me for saving your life, let me take this opportunity to thank you for saving mine."

Every Christmas, Phil sent Paul a Christmas Card and signed each with, *Phil, the guy whose life you saved in the jungle.*

"Morning Lieutenant."

He looked good. Fit, full head of blonde hair, wide smile, white teeth, square jaw. He stood at attention, waiting to be told *at ease*. "Relax Phil. You were discharged nearly 60 years ago."

"Once a soldier, always a soldier." He didn't really believe that and laughed. "How do you feel, Paul?"

"Pretty good given the circumstances. You know, when it's nearly over and they tell you no more can be done, you can ignore every pain, every abdominal discomfort, every new lump. Don't matter. The worst is here, the rest, just window dressing. So, I have some pain, some discomfort and a few new lumps, but other than that, feel pretty good."

"Well, you look pretty good. I'm not a doctor, but if I had to guess, based on what I see, I'd say you have a broken limb, not lung cancer."

"I only wish. But, it is what it is. What's new?"

"Tom Greene died. Leukemia. Probably Agent Orange."

Tom was the Company Commander in Vietnam. A major, a golden oak leaf, now just dead. "Well, if it was Agent Orange, it took its time. Tom must've been nearly 90."

"Ninety-one. On the tennis court until a year ago. I should be so lucky."

"Me too."

When Paul joined the squad, there were 16 members and during his 13 months in country, 14 men replaced those who left for home or died. Of the 30 with whom Paul and Phil served, only eight remained. Five died in Vietnam, one killed himself soon after he returned home, one died of a drug overdose, one in a car accident at age 27, nine of natural causes between the ages of 41 and 65, and five, including Tom Greene, who died of cancers related to Agent Orange. Paul was close, eight would soon be seven.

"If my math is right, there are only eight of us left. And in a short time, after I fall on a grenade, seven."

"Jess Smith is really sick too. So, my friend, you may not get us to seven."

"Six then. Small club."

"You could've been looking at nickel, number five. Without you, I'd have been another in-country casualty."

Paul had remained humble over the almost 60 years following discovery of the trip-wire. Funerals, Celebrations of Life, were for boasting, an opportunity to acknowledge the sacrifices made by the departed, a chance for the dead to take a bow. When others died, when they celebrated monumental birthdays, Paul toasted their accomplishments and tempered talk of his own. Things were now different. It was nearly his time. The time was near. Paul decided he wouldn't wait to bow. "Yup. I think you'd have died but for me. The way the jungle protected the wire, kept it out of sight, it was almost a miracle that I saw it. A breeze likely pushed a branch out of the way and when that branch moved, the sunlight broke through and for a split second, caught the wire, which I saw, because I was at the right place, at the right time. I was lucky to see what I saw, and I think you're right, if I hadn't seen it, you would have died in the jungle."

"You've never said that before."

"Nope. No reason to keep it to myself now."

"Thanks."

"That's not the first time you've said that. I get you appreciate it, but it was my job, and quite frankly, it was dumb luck. I saw that wire, because it was revealed by the sun, which was able to reveal it, because the wind blew. Dumb luck. I was where I needed to be. But I didn't put myself in that position to save you; I was just there. So, without me, you'd be dead, but I'm not a hero, didn't do anything heroic; I was just there and did what anyone else would have done. If I'd have been leading the squad and you were where I was, you'd have saved my life. No question. We were just soldiers, doing our jobs."

Tears filled Phil's eyes and when he closed them to say a silent prayer of thanks, the tears escaped and traveled down Phil's cheeks to his chin where they disappeared into a blonde forest. The forest held no trip wires or attached booby-traps, just blonde hair and tears. "Either way, thank you, Lieutenant."

"Do me a favor?"

"Anything."

"At my funeral, tell war stories. Let 'em all know I was a brave soldier, that I saved your life. Not for me, I'll be gone, but for Mary, for Alyson, Lauren and Randy. Let them know their dad, her husband, was a hero."

"It's the truth and it's always been my plan."

The former soldiers, two heroes, reminisced and talked about Phil's kids, a mailman, a success with regular hours, available overtime and health insurance and a doctor, with unreasonable patients, crazy production requirements and demanding malpractice carriers. They compared Florida notes, Arizona brochures and Texas leaflets and concluded that Phil would be wise to travel to Florida, Texas and Arizona, to shop, before he bought a retirement home. They talked about the upcoming election, Paul diagnosing Republican insanity and Phil predicting rescue by the sane, moderate wing of the party. They pondered the next step, Paul expressing guarded optimism and Phil extolling the absolute belief that good people, especially good people who saved a life, are rewarded in the beyond.

When the conversation circled back to Tom Greene, the recently departed Commander, Phil decided it needed to end. He stood at attention, clicked his heals and saluted his squad leader. "Thank you for everything, Lieutenant. I owe you my life and look forward to our reunion on the other side. Twenty-three good soldiers are waiting for us to join them and when my time comes, I'll be proud to become a member. Thanks, Paul."

About face, left, right, left, right, left, and he was gone.

Before a replacement arrived, Paul grabbed the paper and pen and wrote.

Maybe I saved a life. I'm not so sure. It was out of my control; I simply ate what was provided. I didn't fall on a grenade and destroy my life while saving others, I simply cut a wire that was revealed by the sun and extended the life of my baby brother. He died before he took his first breath, but in Vietnam, with the help of the sun and kismet, I saved his life and resurrected the dead. I'm not a god, wasn't much of a hero, but I did something easy and convenient, yet so important. I made a difference.

*chapter
eighteen*

*W*hen Mary reappeared, Paul told her he wanted to open the bedroom windows, invite the kids in, and have a picnic, *like the old days.*

"I thought the Doctor said, *One at a time.*"

"He may have, but screw it. I'm in charge. What difference will it make? Die an hour earlier? Maybe it'll buoy my spirits and I'll live an extra day. Maybe I die an hour earlier, but am happy as I draw my last breath, because I had a family picnic. The doctor can make recommendations, but I'm the patient, and I'll decide what advice to accept and what advice to reject. I reject *one visitor at a time.* Let's have a picnic."

At 10:30, Lauren and Randy carried the kitchen table over the bedroom threshold and set it next to Paul's bed, close enough that Paul had access to it, when he leaned to his left. Alyson followed, carrying folding chairs that the five family members used for card nights when the children needed help with arithmetic.

A *six, an eight and a jack is 6 plus eight plus ten, 24. Jack, queen and ace, 10 plus 10 plus 11 is 31. Very good, Randy.* When the 30 year old table with 29 year old scratches and a lifetime of spilled juice and milk soaked into its wood grains, and five metal chairs with dents and cushions for bony butts, were in their proper place, Mary unfolded a plastic, red and white checked tablecloth and draped it over the table. The tablecloth had been a wedding gift to Paul and Mary from a spinster aunt who died in the early seventies, and had doubled as a checkerboard when the kids were young and Christmas gifts, including a cardboard checkerboard and plastic pieces, were lost and not found. *King me, Dad.*

While the kids and Mary prepared a picnic lunch, Tom Pertler delivered the mail and good news. "We went to Frank's apartment last night and found a will, or something Frank thought was a will. It was a hand-written, but even though it was just scrawling, he made it clear he had no family and wanted you to have his modest personal property, including his recordings. I talked to Judge Varco this morning and he said he'd sign an order awarding Frank's remains to Mary if you were willing to sign an Affidavit alleging you knew Frank over the last at least 50 years and know he died without family, and believe he nominated you as his only heir in a document he thought was his will."

"You draft it, I'll sign it. Good work Tom. You're a pretty damn good lawyer."

"Not me. Just a practical friend. But I did draft an Affidavit for your signature. It says what Varco wants it to say. If you sign it now, I'll take it to Varco this afternoon and hopefully get the order signed."

"Fast. Almost unbelievable. Excellent!" Paul found the pen he had used minutes earlier, which had rolled down the slope of bedding, into the crevice beneath his light and flat ass, signed the Affidavit and handed it to Tom.

"Varco told me, because no one's followed the law, it's all likely unenforceable, but he doesn't care. He told me his philosophy is, *If it's what* **everyone** *wants and won't be appealed, it's acceptable to him.* Because Frank was alone and had nothing of value, he doesn't think anyone will care or object and as a result, he's willing to sign the order and believes it'll do what you want and likely what Frank wanted."

"Very well-done Tom. After Varco signs the Order, can you bring a copy to the Funeral Home? Please?"

"Will do." Satisfied with his efforts and what they were able to accomplish, he smiled. *Maybe I can be a good lawyer? Huh? Nope. Don't even go there. Haul mail. Keep smiling.* Tom looked at the kitchen table covered with a cloth more appropriately made for a picnic table than a law office, drew in fresh air that entered the room through open windows, smelled fried chicken and baked beans and added, "Time to run. I have mail to deliver and you have a picnic to attend. Enjoy it, my friend."

Tom passed Mary in the doorway and stopped to watch the Thomas children file into the room, carrying picnic goodies. Mary carried a large bowl filled with fried chicken, Lauren a

245

pot full of baked beans, Alyson, paper plates, plastic forks and knives and a diced watermelon and Randy, a 12-pack of Budweiser.

When the picnic table was set and the family seated, Paul spoke. "As always, before we eat, someone's gotta tell a story that makes us laugh, relaxes our bellies and reminds us how special it is to be together. Seeing that I'm the oldest one here, I propose I choose the story and the storyteller. Is that okay?"

Those at the picnic table laughed. They all knew what was coming. Each understood what the story would be and who would tell it. It was Paul's favorite. It was the introduction to seven Christmas dinners, five Thanksgivings and every Father's Day meal since the family decided to dispense with grace and rely on laughter, almost 30 years earlier.

Randy smiled and looked at Lauren. Alyson laughed, covered her mouth to catch chicken she had eaten after removing it from a *Kentucky Fried Chicken* bucket and looked at Lauren. Mary pointed at Lauren, joining the chorus of snickers and prescience. Lauren rolled her eyes. She knew what was coming, it had come so many times before, she almost stood before her name was called. The story was old, cute, but really old and worn. They all knew the punchline, good as it was. There was no surprise, just a tired story. But, given the surroundings, Paul's future and the enthusiasm that always accompanied Paul's request for the story, Lauren smiled.

"Lauren, tell us about Lyndon Johnson's funeral."

Randy opened a beer, took a drink and wiped his smiling mouth. Hungry, impatient and Alyson, Alyson picked up a fork, quickly peeled some skin from a chicken breast and shoveled it into her mouth, where it was devoured by forty bites in thirty seconds, and nodded to Lauren. Mary turned to Lauren, applauded and offered her the stage with a palm extended as if to catch rain from the sky.

Lauren balked. She knew what everyone expected, what they always expected, but this time it was different. It was Lauren's story, but it was *really* her Dad's story. It delighted him and had for half a century. He was there when it was formed. He knew it as well as Lauren, likely better. It was his. "Dad you tell it. I've told it so many times. It delights you and I'd like to sit back and be entertained by you. It's our story and I'd be honored if you told it."

Randy tipped the bottle to his lips and after drinking, tipped it towards his older sister and then his Dad, signaling agreement with Lauren's suggestion. Alyson, being Alyson, told Paul she'd like to hear him tell the story, four times while Randy moved his bottle from the table to his mouth and Mary simply looked at Paul and said, "I agree."

Paul cleared his throat, coughed, coughed again, cleared his throat again and spoke. "Lyndon Johnson, our 36th president died in 1973. Lauren was three-years old. Johnson was a larger than life figure, who became President when a bullet killed President John Fitzgerald Kennedy. Johnson emerged from Kennedy's shadow which had been elongated by his tragic death, and was responsible for important legislation known as the *Great*

Society, that provided help for the unfortunate and equality for minorities. He was a visionary and legislative genius. But, in spite of his domestic genius, he was also responsible for the escalation of the Vietnam War, a war that divided this Country and forced Johnson from office.

"Because Johnson was such an important figure, his death, reviewal and funeral dominated the air waves. For three days, the television screens were fixated on his life and death. Lauren was young, but interested. We watched coverage of President's Johnson's funeral and I explained to Lauren who he was and why his passing was covered as it was.

"She asked me questions and I answered them as well as I could, but I could tell she was pensive about all of it. As Johnson's coffin, covered by an American flag, stood at the front of the church, the cameras focused on it and commentators talked about the man inside, I noticed Lauren curl her upper lip and draw her knees to her chest. I believed she was being frightened by what she saw. She was three, didn't understand life, let alone death. I was afraid that as she looked at the coffin and was told by CBS that a man was in the box, she worried about herself and the possibility that someday, she would be in a box, forever enveloped in a large suitcase.

"I tried to quiet the fears of my little girl. I didn't want her to be afraid of dying and being boxed and buried. I wanted to explain that people have souls and souls escape the body and live eternally in heaven, and as a result, there was no need for her to be afraid. I took her small hand in mine, smiled and offered her comfort. *I want you to know honey, it's just President's*

Johnson's body that's in the box, to which my three-year old daughter responded, *But Daddy, where's his head?"*

"Eat everyone."

Randy offered Paul a Budweiser, but Paul declined. Mary offered Paul a chicken wing, but Paul declined. He wasn't hungry, not thirsty, he just wanted to share time with his family and enjoy the picnic. He smiled.

Lauren stood. She looked at her dad. He was shrinking and the color in his face was disappearing. His lungs crackled as he breathed and he wheezed when he spoke. The student became the teacher, the comforted, the comforter. She smiled. "Dad, it's only your body."

Lauren removed the red smudge on Paul's forehead and kissed him. Paul was tempted to ask Lauren where his head was, but instead, took her hand in his and just smiled.

While Paul watched his family eat and drink, he noticed that each interacted with the others, naturally, playfully and rhythmically, like an instrument whose entries and exits were determined by sheet music and a composer who knew who went where, when and for how long. When the music lagged, when a rest hinted at concert's end, Paul tapped on the lectern and urged the musicians to continue. *Randy, do you remember*...and the aria continued.

Randy was the percussionist. He kept the music moving in time and determined its pace. If another spoke to quickly or misdirected the conversation, Randy politely interrupted, spoke slowly, inviting patience and restraint and returned focus to what had been the source of interest and fun. *But, Alyson, don't you remember Mr. Hadley's most important rule?*

Lauren was the melody, the flute, the saxophone, the cornet, the soprano that gave the wise words, fun words and connective tissue, their beauty. Her voice was strong, always on key, sometimes haunting, sometimes comforting, always melodic. She sang. *He was trying to teach us that life is sometimes challenging, sometimes easy, but always worthwhile.*

Alyson was syncopation, an interruption, a diversion, a cymbal dropped in the back of the music room, a trombone playing the wrong note at the wrong time. When the musical conversation became too comfortable, when its peacefulness bordered on complacency, she disrupted it and required the other musicians to redirect their focus and contribute to a conversation worth having. *That's bullshit. Too easy. There's another explanation and that explanation requires more than yes or no. Figure it out.*

While her musician-children were performing a concerto without notes, Mary reclined her chair, smiled and listened. Appreciative of the concert, recognizing that the notes were struck with precision after years of practice and performing together, the audience, their mother, tapped her foot, hummed along and enjoyed.

Paul's bed was perched above his family, closer to the heavens. He wanted to be at the table below, amongst them, jawing, eating, drinking, making music, having fun, but the side-rails keep the sick in bed and he was sick. He closed his eyes, joined Mary in the audience, and let the music sweep him away....

"What do you think, Dad?"

Asked to perform, Paul opened his eyes and admitted he had been away and didn't understand the question. "Sorry, I didn't get the question. Ask again, please." Because the question was asked by Alyson, Paul added, "And do so slowly, please."

"Randy believes Frank died alone and that makes his life less significant. Lauren believes Frank touched lives in other ways and his life was as significant as he wanted it to be and I don't think it makes any difference whatsoever, he's gone, he did what he did, left what he left, found what he's going to find and it doesn't matter anymore."

Randy directed and corrected his younger sister. "Slow down, it's hard to understand what you're saying. I didn't say his life was insignificant. I said, as a parent, he would have touched more lives in a more significant manner and as a result, his life would have had *more* impact."

"What I really said was, Frank was a wonderful man, and did what he was destined to do. He was odd, but that's okay, odd people have a special place. Because he was different, it was hard for him to find a mate and if he had, it would have been difficult for him to raise children in a conformist society. He did what he loved, something others wouldn't do, and as a result filled gaps and made people smile for odd reasons, in odd ways. His life wasn't Lauren rich, Randy rich or Alyson rich, but it was

Frank rich and that's all he could have asked for." Lauren rested her flute on her lap and waited for the cymbal to drop. And it did.

"Who cares? He's dead. His contribution has been made. *You da man* is over. Fun? Okay. Rich? Who knows. Worthwhile. I don't care."

Mary smiled.

Alyson asked again. "What do you think, Dad?"

"I think you're all right. It depends on your perspective. I'm not sure. What I do know is that you all have different opinions, and all of your opinions are considerate and kind. No one is suggesting Frank was a loser. No one is suggesting he was worthless. He was odd, but he was kind. You all recognize his contribution; you just disagree on its impact. Just don't have this same conversation in a week or two when talking about me. There should be no disagreement. My impact has been substantial and overwhelmingly positive. If you disagree, I ask you to look at the evidence presented in this room. I'm proud of all of you."

The drummer, the vocalist, the well-intentioned artist who dropped the cymbal while the band played on, and the audience, all smiled and in unison said, "Thanks, Dad." And Paul smiled.

The picnickers sat at the table and chatted. They drank beer, picked at chicken bones and remembered picnics in parks, by the lakeshore and under summer skies. They remembered swings as much larger and able to go much higher than they really had. They remembered horseshoe pits and many more ringers than were actually thrown. The lake water of their memory was colder than it really was in June and warmer than it really was in August, and the winds and rain of a storm that chased them from a picnic table, leaving potato salad, watermelon and sandwiches on a green table whose paint was pocked by the sun, were stronger and more substantial, as they remembered, than those of the storm that had really chased them to their car in 1986. In their collective memory, everything was bigger, colder, stronger, hotter, more disruptive and more perfect than it had really been. It was natural; it was what time does, distorts in favor of miraculous.

Paul remembered, but because his time was short, the time that passed had not distorted his reality. He remembered the water as lukewarm in both June and August and the storm as inconvenient, not cataclysmic. It was all very clear, as was his perception of the picnickers. *Good, honest, loving, sweet, courageous, enthusiastic, kind.* Although he wished he could remain, to create more memories, memories that likely would be distorted when Alyson, Lauren or Randy succeeded him to a bed with side-rails, distortions discussed when they gathered to say *Goodbye* again, he was glad they had done what had been done, and that their memories were ones that made them happy. They made him happy as well. *Thank God for family. Thank God for my family.*

chapter
nineteen

Paul closed his eyes and when they opened, the table covered by the red and white checkerboard, the dented chairs, the chicken, beans, watermelon and beer and his family were gone. Belle sat in the only chair that remained, a chair that reclined and provided lumbar support, watching a muted television. "What'cha watching?"

Belle pushed a button and the television screen turned black. She looked at Paul and answered the question he asked. "You."

"You can watch television. I don't care. Multi-task as Mary says. Watch me, watch T.V. Or find something that interests me and then watch me watch T.V."

"Maybe later. Unless there's something you want to watch."

"Nope."

"Ron was here and left your mail. He said the Judge signed the Order and he got a copy to the mortuary. They told him they'd cremate Frank's remains and have them delivered to you."

"Belle, can you ask Mary to call the mortuary and tell them to put Frank in a wood urn before delivering them to me. Light colored wood if possible."

"I can call them. If I've got to say it once, might as well say it to the source."

"Thanks. I didn't know if I could ask you to do that. It's probably not in the job description."

Belle chuckled, surveyed a list in her mind and said, "I've done lots that's not in the job description. I painted a bathroom for a woman with congenital heart failure and stopped a leak in a cancer patient's toilet. I sang to a child born with a compromised immune system and shined the shoes of an elderly gentleman who asked that I help prepare him for his meeting with St. Peter. So, a telephone call? Not in the job description, but not out of bounds. Happy to help in any way I can."

As Belle made a note to herself, Paul fanned through his mail. Junk and cards. He tossed the junk into a wastebasket alongside the bed and marked the cards received with his pen. *407, 408, 409, 410, 411, 412, 413, 414.* A light day.

When he was first diagnosed and his condition publicized on *Caring Bridge*, Paul was inundated with *Get Well* cards. Every day, he received a stack of cards. After a week, he asked Mary how many cards she thought he had received, and after she guessed, Paul guessed. *75. 104.* After recording their guesses on an imaginary recorder, Paul asked for the pile of cards on the kitchen table and counted them. *108. I win.* Since then, he numbered every card received, just in case Mary decided to resurrect the competition.

The flavor of the cards had changed. The cards he first received were cute, loud and colorful. Talking ducks, puppies, wrinkled people on a golf course, stick people who spoke in bubbles with words written in cursive, turtles without their shells, kittens and striped and spotted fish in an aquarium. The messages were uplifting, comical and cute. *Tell the quack to administer the right medicine and we'll see you in the pond. Heard about the ruff times; get well soon. Sorry you're over par; see the swing doctor and make a tee-time. Follow doctors' orders and restore purr-rrr-fection. Shed your shell, beat your bug and get well. Sorry you've stumbled into the water, but we all know you'll do swimmingly well.*

When treatment didn't fix him, when messages Mary posted on Paul's *Caring Bridge* site changed from *We're optimistic and The fight has just begun,* to *The focus is now on comfort* and *Some fights are worth waging, even though victory is unattainable,* the cards changed. 288 was white, blue, red and whacky and 289 was simply white and somber, as were all those that followed. *As you complete your journey, may peace be your companion. Surround yourself with family; surround yourself with comfort. ....and God smiled.*

He received a card from a man he successfully prosecuted in 1968, a man who had served nine years in prison and hadn't seen or talked to Paul since sentencing. Randy's class sent a card, as did Frank, two days before he died. Fourteen classmates from Anoka Class of '57, sent well-wishes through the mail and cards arrived from Australia, Egypt, Paraguay, Saudi Arabia, Bosnia, Sweden, Greenland and Russia. Eight people who signed cards, died while Paul received treatment and laid in hospice, and two were diagnosed with lung cancer after sending a card and were receiving the same treatments that failed Paul. Paul sent a card to those who suffered as he had. The cards Paul sent were inspired by experience. He knew where they were and likely, where they would be. The cards Paul sent, were somber and white.

Two of the cards Paul received on the day Belle agreed to call the mortuary, numbers 408 and 412, were the same and sent from lawyers with whom Paul had cases. The cards were the same, the lawyers, extremely different. Steve Frank was conciliatory and soft-spoken, a worthy adversary more interested in a fair settlement than a trial. Lon Jones was loud, offensive and verbose, a worthy adversary more interested in trial than any kind of settlement. Both men were honest, hard-working and competent, and Paul learned when he opened their cards, religious. *May the grace of Jesus Christ, Lord and Savior, provide you peace.*

Sometimes Paul opened the cards, read them, closed his eyes, reflected on the messages conveyed and was filled with appreciation for the sender and the printed and written words, but sometimes, he tore open the envelope, opened the card and read only the name of the sender, ignoring the oftentimes pompous, patronizing and puritanical message written by a healthy 25 year old with a Bachelor's degree in English, in a Hallmark office in Kansas City, Missouri. *Tripe. Hollow. Insincere. Materialistic.*

The cards were too expensive, their messages forgettable, not worth the investment. Long before it was fashionable, he and

Mary picked out Valentine's cards for one another, while they were together at Target, and read them and returned them to the rack. With the eight dollars saved, they drank wine with their Valentine's dinner.

The cards that pleased Paul most, the ones that he invariably read from beginning to end, were the cards that contained no pre-printed message from the manufacturer in the card's bowels. If Paul opened a card, discovered that the message was created by the sender, that the words were written by the sender and printed with the aid of a pen, he read all that was written. He was touched by the effort. People older than Paul scrawled well wishes with cramped hands made evident by almost illegible letters pocked with tremble marks and the inability to allow the pen to comfortably cruise up and down and across the page. Authors without skill or the vaguest idea of punctuation, coined warm greetings that were difficult if not impossible to understand. It didn't matter the skill of the wordsmith or the beauty of the penmanship, the effort was clear and *it* was the message Paul received. They cared enough to try, understanding their attempt was a stick-figure drawing in an art gallery or a misfit story in a collection of Shakespearean works. Humbled, they wrote from their hearts and Paul heard them say, *I love you, get well.*

Number 414 was written by a voice from 1994. Dying, it appeared, resurrected relationships long dead. It was signed by Roy Anderson. The return address was Stillwater Correctional Facility, Stillwater, MN.

Even here, we get the local news. I was told you are sick and in hospice. I hope the news was inaccurate, but if not, I pray for a peaceful passage to the glorious heavens painted and maintained by a merciful God. Semper Fi. Roy A.

Paul smiled and gave the *Little Marine* credit for not holding a grudge. Paul remembered Roy A as the *Little Marine*. The investigators never referred to him as Roy Anderson, Mr. Anderson, the suspect or defendant, outside of the courtroom or during discussions, they always called him the *Little Marine*. Twice during the trial, in chambers, the Judge called him the *Little Marine* and television scrawls and headlines referred to him as Roy Anderson, the *Diminutive Marine*. *Diminutive* was too many syllables, to Paul, he'd always be the *Little Marine*.

Five-foot-five-inches of Marine spit and polish, religious arrogance, anger, intolerance. The *Little Marine* was a low-level military hero. He received a Purple Heart and served two tours of duty in Vietnam. Some suggested he suffered from *Little Man's Disease*, others believed he was a big man with a large heart in a small body. His critics alleged he carried a gun in Southeast Asia, because it added five inches to his rather short skeleton and his supporters lauded him for bravery and a willingness to step into danger for his Country. Paul didn't know him in Vietnam, didn't choose a side in the motive argument, but when he thought of him, he smiled and said, the *Little Marine*.

The *Little Marine* was charged with three counts of murder in 1993. One of the victims was his 17 year old daughter. He admitted pulling the trigger, admitted he intended to kill the victims, talked freely to investigators who he thought would *understand*, quoted the Bible, the Uniform Code of Military Justice and his drill sergeant and demanded and received a jury trial.

He was convicted of first degree murder after an hour of jury deliberations.

Paul was a member of the prosecution team. He sat at counsel table during the trial, gave the State's opening statement, questioned two of the investigators and helped the County Attorney, the face of the State's team, with his closing argument. Although two lawyers sat at the State's table, only one was necessary. Even though three prosecutors researched the law and made arguments to the Judge, none were necessary. It wasn't a difficult case that invited complicated legal arguments; it wasn't an exercise in plotting, planning and patience, designed to illicit damning testimony from reams of denials and distortions. It was simple, easier than a court trial designed to determine if a driver exceeded the speed limit. The facts were uncontroverted. It was a battle of philosophies and the law was largely irrelevant.

The *Little Marine* was an absolutist. He was absolutely right, about everything. Ask him and he told you. *I'm right.* When logic and fact entered the conversation, and suggested the *Little Marine* was wrong, he quoted the Bible and relied on twisted interpretations and inspiration he claimed, came directly from God.

On March 8, 1993, while watching television, the *Little Marine* heard someone rattle the handle of his back door. Rather than call the police or leave his residence through the front door, Anderson opened a metal locker that doubled as a coffee table and removed a rifle he had modified so that it could empty a 25-bullet clip in seconds. He turned the rocking chair on which he sat so it faced the back door, turned off the rifle's safety, took a drink of beer, and waited. As he told the jury, he smiled as he waited.

When a young man wearing black walked over the threshold into Anderson's home, Anderson cleared his throat loudly, and the intruder turned and ran from the *Little Marine's* residence. Anderson calmly walked to the open back door, stepped onto the stoop, watched three people run away, raised his rifle to his shoulder, pulled the trigger, discharged 25 bullets and killed three people. The Little Marine didn't check on his victims, but instead, walked into the house, finished his beer, removed his empty clip from his rifle, cleaned his weapon, returned the rifle to the metal box and then called the police.

Two hours after the police arrived, Roy Anderson was hand-cuffed and led from his home to a police cruiser. As he walked towards the car with flashing red lights, for the first time, he looked at his victims, illuminated by search lights and bloodied by bullets, and saw he had killed his daughter.

The *Little Marine* pleaded not guilty and demanded a jury trial. After the State rested its case and Anderson and his court appointed attorney argued about the wisdom of Anderson taking the stand and providing testimony, Anderson discharged his attorney and represented himself through the conclusion of the trial. He took the stand and said,

*May the grace of God and his almighty son, Jesus Christ, guide and forgive me. **Irregardless** of how the evidence has described me, I killed my daughter and feel bad about that. I wish she was here, but believe she's in a better place.*

*So far, this trial has been all about what I did. It should be about more. It should be about why I did what I did. **Irregardless***

of what the prosecutors say, I'm a good American and didn't do anything wrong. I know three kids are dead, but that's not the point.

What is the point? The point is, President Clinton wants to take my guns. I have the constitutional right to own guns and liberals want to take that right away. The Second Amendment of our United States Constitution says I have the right to bear arms. I fought for that and liberals want to take that right away. No one says the Pledge of Allegiance in Schools anymore. Can't say a prayer in schools to start the day and God forbid if we required kids to learn about how the world was really created. It's in the Bible, but don't say it too loud, or they'll arrest you and charge with some crime. I know. Look at me.

Irregardless *of what they say, I did nothing wrong, but exercise my God given, Constitutional rights. A man's house is his castle. Read the Bible. A man has the right to protect his castle from the seedier elements and the Constitution of these United States, says I can do that with guns. When guns are outlawed, only the criminals will have guns, and then, I'm the one who's dead. Is that fair? Is that right? They kill babies and want to deny me the right to defend my home. Is that right? I don't think so.*

Irregardless *of what prosecutors say, I'm not a bad guy. I served in Vietnam two times and wear a Purple Heart. I own lots of guns, some modified to do what I want them to do, but does that make me bad? No. It makes me a God fearing, believer in the Second Amendment.*

*The cops said I should have let the intruders leave. They were running away, just let them go. That's an **irregardless** argument.*

I didn't know if they'd come back. I have a God given right to feel safe in my own home and when that kid rattled the door and stepped into my house, he took that away. I had a right to make sure that it wouldn't happen again. I did what I needed to do.

When the *Little Marine* stopped talking and looked at the Judge, signaling that he had said all he intended to say, the Judge asked the County Attorney if he had questions for Mr. Anderson. Cross examination is designed to obtain testimony favorable to the questioner's position, and because the *Little Marine* had said everything the prosecution could have hoped for, and much, much more, Paul's boss smiled without smiling and said, "No questions, Your Honor."

An hour after being instructed, the Jury returned to the courtroom and pronounced its verdicts. *Guilty. Guilty. Guilty.* At sentencing, the *Little Marine* was sentenced to three consecutive life in prison terms. After pronouncing his sentence, as an afterthought, the Judge added, "You will remain in prison until your daughter can confront you and damn you for your arrogance."

Paul wasn't an advocate for gun control, nor was he a proponent of guns rights. His involvement in the case of the *Little Marine* didn't change his opinion; he remained a centrist. He didn't understand the absolutists on either side. When kids were killed, in school, in Colorado and New York, he wondered about the wisdom of making semi-automatic weapons available to the deranged, thought *something* should be done, but said little, knowing his words would fuel anger and exaggerate intractability. He had fought his guns rights fight. He wasn't any longer interested.

Semper fi. Roy A. (Inmate No. 99456). When Paul finished reading number 414 and dropped it on the stack of cards, Belle returned to Paul's prison. She had completed her mission. "Frank will be here tomorrow morning."

"Good. Then I'll have someone to talk to in the middle of the night when I can't sleep."

Paul wasn't sure if Frank remained largely as he was when he played Paul a recording less than 48 hours earlier or had been transformed to ashes. He remembered others referring to Frank as *cremated,* but wasn't certain the transformation was complete. If his body awaited the crematorium, he'd be stiffer and the color would have disappeared from his face. If he hadn't met the fire, Paul would have been able to pick him out of a line-up of dead guys who were the same height and weight as Frank. He'd know the hairline, the nose, the weak chin, large eyes and tiny ears. He'd identify Frank instantly. If he hadn't been cremated. Yet.

Paul pictured Frank's body on a steel gurney. No clothes, no jewelry, no smile. The sheet had been removed. No need for humility. He's dead and undertakers, embalmers, mortuary science students and crematorium owners have no interest in what the sheet had hidden and what it revealed when it was pulled from the corpse. The gurney's wheels squeak as the undertaker pushes Frank towards the oven. Is the undertaker smoking? Chewing gum? When he greets mourners on the floor above, the floor with flowers, carpet, white oak, caskets, an altar and Guest Books, he wears a black suit and tie and black leather shoes. When he pushes Frank toward the fire, is he wearing shorts, a tee-shirt and tennis shoes? Is he like the rest of us, does the presence of the dead make him feel creepy, mortal? When he transfers Frank from the gurney to the crematorium, does he struggle with the dead weight, does he call for help, does he crank a lever that lowers Frank's feet and raises his head, so that he slips from the steel bed into the fire pit? Does Frank hear the door close? When the man who wears suits upstairs and shorts downstairs in the basement without carpet, pushes the button and the flames burn dead flesh, does Frank feel the heat?

"Penny for your thoughts."

Mary's words pulled Paul from the mortuary to the hospice. Not a long trip. "Just thinking about Frank. Belle says he'll be here tomorrow."

"See. It could be worse."

"Maybe. I've asked myself if it's better to have time to say *Goodbye* and time to fret dying or go without notice. My way or Frank's way? I'm glad I'm still alive, wouldn't trade with Frank, but he didn't suffer, didn't fret. He sat down and, boom, it was over. Quick. Clean. No hassles. No hospice."

"Well, I agree with you. I'm glad that you're still alive. I'm better off that you're still here. And if you love life, you want to live it as long as possible, unless you're in such pain that it can't be enjoyed. And I think meds are managing your pain. You picnicked with your family. Doesn't get any better than that."

Paul framed the mental picture he had taken at the picnic. Everyone was happy, everyone smiled, everyone shared happy memories, everyone laughed and shielded themselves from the sun's harsh rays with a roof. "It was fun. At my stage in life, observation is as important as participation. I no longer need to be the center of attention. My opinions aren't as important as they once were. I don't have an agenda to pursue. So, I can sit back and observe and appreciate. What I saw, I liked. We did a good job. Those are pretty good kids."

"Kids? Lauren's closer to fifty than forty and nobody needs to teach Randy or Alyson how to ride a bike or drive a car. They're pretty good people who happen to be our kids. And I agree, when you look at who they have become, we did a good job."

Paul grinned and wiped a tear from his cheek. When Mary saw that he was emotional, she asked, "What's wrong?"

"Nothing. Something's right. It was a tear of joy." He wiped another away. "When I was young and the kids were really young, when I struggled as a parent, when I second guessed decisions I made or a parenting tool I employed, and wondered if I was contributing to a catastrophe or smash hit, I told myself, *Keep trying, do the best you can, and when you're old and dying, maybe you can evaluate your skills by looking at what you leave behind.* Well, I'm old and dying and yesterday, during the picnic, I evaluated my skills by looking at what I was leaving behind. I must've been skillful. I'm leaving behind wonderful kids. I'm proud of them, but I'm also proud of my contribution. My decisions must've been the right ones and the parenting tools I employed, must've worked. They're good kids. We did do a hell of a job."

chapter twenty

Paul stood over the deep sink and breathed hot steam into the far reaches of his lungs. He needed to blink his eyes every couple of seconds, or they became clouded with evaporated hot water and he was unable to see. The paper hat he wore, soaked with perspiration and steam, began to split at the seams and fall over his forehead and cover his eyes and block his vision. He lifted the cap five times so he could better see the sink, but when it slipped for a sixth time, he pulled it from his head, crumpled it into a wet paper ball and tossed it into the garbage with soiled napkins, ketchup soaked, partially eaten hamburger buns, runny, sticky, unruly egg yolks, cold French fries, shredded toothpicks and cigarette butts soaked in soda, coffee or maple syrup. As he scrubbed a plate corroded with dried egg yolk, his Dad dropped a large plastic tub of dirty dishes on the counter next to the sink and barked, "Pick up the pace. We're almost out of forks."

School had been cancelled and Paul celebrated the surprise by shoveling 18-inches of snow from the driveway. The driveway wasn't long or wide, but wind made his task difficult. He couldn't throw the snow, because a 25-mile an hour wind grabbed what was tossed to the air and returned it to the driveway, so he filled his shovel, walked to the edge of the pavement, and dropped his load on snow covered grass. Over and over and over again. When the driveway was clean, he shoveled a path from the detached garage to the back door of his parents' house and after removing his bunny boots, sat on the couch and took a deep, relaxing breath. Before he could exhale, the phone rang.

"Paul?"

"Yeah."

"You need to come to the restaurant. I need you."

"Huh?"

"Two waitresses and the dishwasher called. They can't get out of their driveways. The snow. Every truck with a plow is out and they all want coffee and something to eat. They're here. I can't keep up. I need help."

"But Dad, how do I get there?"

"Don't know. I've got to go. Thanks."

Paul sat on the couch, exhaled the breath he had taken before he answered his Dad's call, put his bunny boots on cold feet, zipped his parka, pulled a stocking cap over his ears and covered his mitts with choppers. As he stepped into the cold wind, he turned and shouted to his mother, who baked when it snowed, "I'm going to the restaurant to help Dad."

The restaurant was two-miles from home. It was west of town and the 25-mile an hour wind was in his face, chilling his cheeks and delaying his progress. He leaned into the wind, hunched his shoulders, found tracks in the snow left by trucks, and walked. And walked. And walked.

Forty minutes after he left the warmth of his home, Paul walked into the warmth of *Hi-Ten Café*. While he kicked snow from his frozen boots and removed his hat and unzipped his coat, revealing pink cheeks, his Dad flashed by and said, "What took you? I need you in the scullery."

The sink was deep and full. Plastic tubs filled with dirty dishes lined the long counter and like his Dad, waited for Paul. Paul arrived after the lunch rush and emptied all the tubs and cleaned all the plates, bowls, cups, glasses and silverware, just before the supper crowd arrived. By eight o-clock, the restaurant was nearly empty and all of the dinnerware was cleaned and stacked, ready for the next day.

Sitting at the counter, eating a burger and waiting for his Dad to finish his bookwork and count his money, Paul smiled, proud of his accomplishments. *Shovel, walk, wash and survive. Not bad for a teen. Not bad for 13.*

When he opened his eyes, resting against side rails cushioned by a pillow, Paul remembered his dream. Some he remembered, some he forgot. The dream of snow, shoveling, walking and washing dishes, he remembered. It was recurrent. Sixty-two years after snow cancelled school, he relived the day in dreams. He wasn't certain how much of what he remembered was true, how much was fiction, embellished by time and self-aggrandizement, but the memory was clear and visited him often. He pushed the button, raising his head and wrote.

Does it matter if I walked two miles over snow covered roads, into 25-mile an-hour winds, to help my Dad? What if the snow depth was six-inches as opposed to 18? What if the wind was from the east, at my back, and not 25-miles an-hour, but rather 10? And if my Mom drove me to the restaurant, what difference does it make? If the snow kept people off the roads, so that the restaurant was empty, not full and the dirty dishes non-existent, so what?

What matters now is not the truth, but what I remember the truth to be or what my Dad remembered as the truth when he reflected on his short life, as it ended. The distortions, if there are distortions, are designed to make me happy, to make my life appear to be more than it was, to make my Dad happy when he needed recollections to fend off impending loneliness.

I couldn't choose my parents, the place of my birth or when it occurred, but I can choose to remember it as I wish. While imprisoned in a broken body, unable to leave my bed and make more memories, I can remember things as I wish. What does it matter?

I was born in Neverland. My father was a prince, my mother, Cinderella. When it snowed in 1953, I crawled 10 miles over three feet of snow, into 40 mile an hour winds and saved my dad from evil. And we lived happily ever after.

Paul smiled. His life was truly magical.

Mary walked into Paul's room and grinned. She carried something in addition to her smile. "Good morning." She tilted her forehead toward what she carried and asked, "Guess what I have here?"

It was a brown box, with brass hinges and a brass latch. It was the size of two shoe boxes, blonde, polished, simple and elegant. A small brass nameplate adorned the top of the box, but Paul was unable to read the letters. He didn't need to, he knew what they said. "Good morning, Frank."

"Where do you want him?"

"Where do you think he'll be most comfortable?"

"I don't think it makes a difference to Frank."

"Will you say that about me in a few days or weeks?"

"If you're in a box, probably."

Paul looked at his frail, disappearing hands, his uncovered, long, yellowing toes with curling nails, pulled loose skin from his forearm, expecting it to snap back when released, released it and watched it hang low, without elasticity, unable to return to muscle and bone, frowned and said, "I'm close to the box now. Not much left." When he looked at what remained of Frank, when he considered the options, when he remembered he was still here, still breathing, still talking, still writing, still picnicking, he smiled. "Put him on the dresser, facing the television. If he gets bored, he can watch re-runs of *Seinfeld*."

"I think he preferred golf."

"Only if he had been there and had been able to get in a *You da Man*. He once told me George Costanza and Eddie Haskell were television's two greatest characters. Eddie, because he was so pleasantly smarmy, and George, because he was what Frank always wanted to be, without purpose, without direction, without boundaries."

"Wanted to be? Wasn't Frank without direction, purpose and boundaries?"

"Not according to Frank. He was in the business of recording history. Frank thought he was doing something important. Seems like people either believe they contribute nothing of importance or that their contributions are immense and unequaled. Frank was in the latter category. Like Trump."

When her grandfather died young, when Mary was seven, Mary asked her mother if he died because he was so mean. Mary's mother looked to see if anyone had heard, hushed her and whispered, *Don't ever speak unkind of the dead. Remember them as happy, good people. Say only kind things about them. Maybe they're listening.* Mary was a good learner and once learned, her lessons weren't forgotten. "Frank was a nice man. He can rest comfortably on the dresser and hopefully, he's resting comfortably in the hereafter."

"Yeah, like Trump. *You da man. You're fired.* Equally important. Equally nonsensical. I loved Frank, but he was behind Trump. Thought he would shake things up. *Make America Great Again.*

Sure, you blowhard." Paul look sheepishly at the blonde box and added, "That was directed at Trump, not Frank."

Defending the dead, speaking kindly of the departed, remembering her mother's words, Mary added. "Frank would've come around. Trump's entertainment. He's not serious. If he is, he's failing miserably. Frank would've figured that out."

"I hope so, but we'll ever know. He won't cast a ballot now." Looking to the dresser, to the right of the television screen, at a blonde box, "Will you, Frank?" Frank didn't answer, so Paul continued, uninterrupted. "You have more faith in people than I do. I watch that clown on television. He gives speeches and says nothing. He's inarticulate. Knows nothing about the issues. He blabbers and stumbles and the big crowds that gather to watch him make a fool out of himself, don't understand that he's an idiot, incapable of rational thought. They cheer his every stumble. I hope it's just people turning out to see a celebrity and it goes no further. If it does, watch out."

Trump wasn't dead. Mary's mother hadn't suggested he be protected. Mary was free to say what she believed true about the living, about Trump. "He's a dope with a bad haircut. He's feasting on bigotry. It can't last long."

Mary and Paul looked at Frank. They wanted confirmation, to be told by a mystic that they were right, that Trump had no chance, that he would fade with September warmth, but Frank didn't move, didn't speak.

Mary brushed Paul's hair with her fingers, scowled at the lock that wouldn't mind, the graying incorrigible, unreasonable strands, and suggested talk of politics end. "Enough Trump. Keep talking about him, my heart might sputter and I'll be in hospice with you. The bed's not big enough for two."

Paul grinned. "I'll make room." Remembering what he saw and felt when he last checked under his pajamas, he tempered his thoughts and ultimately, his words. "A cuddle is all I could give at this point. But, I'll make room."

Mary got it. She understood. She read articles about men and women exercising passions into the late eighties, but had happily accepted celibacy at 65. It was easier. No need for suggestive underwear, bedside lube or convoluted explanations or apologies when it didn't work. It had been wonderful for 40 years, but it was no more. They didn't talk about it; had never acknowledged its disappearance. It left and they left it at that. "In your dreams."

Paul lifted the stubborn lock of hair and pulled it to the top of his head and when he removed his hand, it stubbornly fell to his forehead. "Do you want me to get a scissors and get rid of it?"

"No. Gotta look my best. If it bugs me, you can plaster it with gel and put it wherever you want. It won't move then."

Mary moved sheets, tossed used tissues into the wastebasket and adjusted the rolling table so that it was near Paul and parallel to the bed-rails. She filled a cup with ice and water, covered it with a lid and punctured the lid with a straw and set it on the table, within Paul's reach. She placed her hands on her hips, surveyed the fruits of her labors and said, "Richie is here. Want me to send him in?"

"Sure."

Paul Richmond, Richie, was a kid who moved to Anoka in fifth grade. Paul sat behind him in Mrs. Ottenstroer's class. Richie was quiet, studious, friendless. At recess, while the other boys played baseball, dodge ball, tag or huddled and whispered about girls, Richie stood alone, watching. It was his third sixth grade classroom, and he had learned it was easier to stay to himself than make friends he would likely discard in months.

Richie had lived in nine foster homes and the Richmond home in Anoka was his tenth. His biological parents were 14 and 15 when Richie was born, and although they tried to keep and raise him, because they were young and without skill or resources, and their parents who believed Jesus would not understand childbirth to an unmarried couple, didn't support their decision to raise a child as an unmarried couple or Richie, who they recognized as a consequence of sinful conduct, not a kid, Family Services took him from his parents and placed him in foster home after foster home after foster home.

The Richmonds were in their fifties and had concluded that after twenty-years of unprotected, childless sex, they were not likely to give birth to a baby, so applied for and received a foster care license. Richie was placed in their home in April, 1952.

Richie was compliant, cold. Too many homes, too many foster parents. He expected he would be in Anoka until summer and move on. He always had. Because he suspected his stay with the Richmonds would be short, he didn't invest. They were kind, nice, made Richie good meals and provided him with a warm home, robustly hugged him while his arms dispassionately dangled at his sides, but Richie knew, like all the others, they'd soon be gone, so he invested little.

When he was placed in his first foster home, he was too young to know. When he was placed in his third home, he was four-years-old, the same age as his foster brother. They played, fought, bonded. When Richie's belongings were packed and he was moved to number four, he missed his brother, and at night, cried.

Number five was idyllic. He was the fourth child in the home. They ate together, played together, made plans together. When Richie laid in bed at night, he said prayers and thanked God for his family. When he was moved to home number six, he stopped dreaming, stopped thanking God and stopped investing.

Seven, eight and nine were adequate. Father figure. Mother figure. Four walls, a roof, a bed and food. And a car and the help needed to move him out and down the road.

When he was enrolled in Washington Elementary, the Richmonds told his teacher he would finish the school year at Washington and that, to the best of their knowledge, he was where he should have been academically. Tolerating number ten and dreading number eleven, Richie stood apart from the other boys on the playground and watched.

On a hot summer night in August, 1952, Anne Richmond told Richie that she and her husband Don, had decided they would adopt Richie. She asked if that would be okay with Richie and he said, *Sure*. He wasn't enthusiastic, not emotionally committed, just tired of moving. *They're okay and this is okay. Beats number eleven.*

On the first day of sixth grade, Paul learned he was assigned to Mrs. Leonard's class. Cliff was in the class, as was Richie. When they finished lunch, and headed to the playground for recess, Paul asked Richie if he'd ever played baseball, and when he said he had, Paul said, *You're on my team. Come on.*

Richie became an odd member of the group. Odd, not repulsive. Odd, not bad. Odd, just different. Nothing excited Richie. He never screamed, shouted, jumped in place, laughed uncontrollably, trembled from nervousness or cried. When others laughed, he smiled. When others screamed, he held a small lump in his throat and when it passed, softly said, *Wow.* When others cried, he looked away. In eighth grade, North Street won the City Baseball Championship for the first time in 42 years when Richie hit a two-run homerun in the bottom of the ninth, and when he stepped on home-plate to record the winning run, he was swamped with screaming, jumping 13 year olds, and he just smiled and offered a handshake.

That same summer, Richie and Paul were walking home from the bowling alley, where they played pinball and pool, when a car pulled to the curb and the driver, a middle-aged man, with a belly but no hair, with blue eyes, but no chin, rolled down the window and said, "Hey, Paul."

Paul didn't know the man and had no idea how he knew him, but when Richie answered, Paul remembered Richie's real name was Paul, and it was Richie to whom the driver had offered his greeting.

Richie nodded at the man, but kept walking. When the car moved forward and stopped adjacent to the boys for the second time, the driver spoke again. "It's been a long time. Do you live here now?"

Richie stopped, put his hands on his hips, bent at the waist so that he could see into the car and speak to the driver, face-to-face. "Yeah, I live here. What do you want?"

"I thought maybe you'd like to see Steve."

Richie perked up and smiled. "Where is he?"

"Not far from here. He's playing in a baseball tournament in Coon Rapids. I can take you there if you want. I'll bring you back later."

Richie withdrew his head from the car's interior, stood tall and looking right, left, over the car and behind it, surveyed his surroundings. He dropped his hands from his hips and rubbed his quads. He bent over, looked in the car again, said nothing and stood straight and mumbled to himself. As he considered his options, he motioned Paul to come closer and when he did, he said, "This guy was a foster parent. I lived with him for about a year. Steve was another kid who lived there. I thought Steve was gone too, but I guess I was wrong."

Richie bent over, looked in the car and asked, "You sure Steve's in Coon Rapids?"

"Why would I lie about that."

Richie looked away from the man in the car and toward Paul. He whispered. "Steve and I were pretty close. When I was removed from the house, it all happened pretty fast and I never understood what happened. But, I always liked Steve. He was like a brother. I'd like to see him and see how he's doing."

"Let's go kid. Come or don't come. It's up to you, but I've got to get out of here. I'm blocking the road." He pulled the shift knob toward the back seat, dropping the transmission from neutral to drive, and stood on the brakes, keeping the car in position next to Richie. He lifted his foot from the brake and the car moved forward about a foot, letting Richie know a quick decision was in order.

Richie shuffled forward, leaned into the car, leaned out, got tall, looked around surveying the area for obstacles to his rendezvous with Steve, bent down and said, "Okay. I'm coming."

Richie leaned out of the car and to Paul said, "I won't be long. If my parents start looking for me, tell them you don't know where I am. Adoption's a strange thing. They're good people. I don't want them to think I'm choosing some step-parent over them. So, don't tell them. I don't want to hurt their feelings."

Richie jumped in the car and they drove away, leaving Paul alone and confused, nearly guilty, on the side of the road. When Paul walked home, through the door, and turned on the television, it was 3:30.

At 5:30, Richie's mom called Paul and asked if he knew where Richie was. Paul said, *No*. The next morning, Paul called Richie and was told by Richie's mom that he was in the hospital and would be there for a few days. When Paul asked if he could visit him, Richie's mom said, *No*.

Something in Richie's mom's voice lead Paul to believe she didn't want him to ask *What happened?*, so he didn't ask. When he saw Richie ten days later, he was quiet, reserved and reluctant to share. He smiled, but the smile was modest, insincere and quick to come and go. He whistled, not a tune, but rather impatiently to summon a tardy friend. He spoke, but said little. Paul didn't ask him directly, but he gave Richie every opportunity to explain. *Wow man. Did they treat you okay in the hospital? How you feeling man? You're quiet buddy, are you all right?*

Richie never offered an explanation and Paul was either too timid or too respectful to ask. Two weeks after Richie was released from the hospital, Paul overheard his Mom and Dad whisper details they wanted to hide from Paul.

What an animal.

Who?

The guy who sexually assaulted Richie. Can you imagine? Sick bastard.

Richie's mom said he lost his foster care license because he was abusing teen-aged boys and went to prison. Two weeks out, and he came looking for Richie. Poor kid.

When he gets out of the hospital, I'm guessing he'll return to prison.

A waste of money, housing him in prison. Richie should have killed him. He hit him once with a shovel and knocked him out. Should have hit him a few more times and killed him.

Poor kid has enough to carry with him. Killing him would've added to his burden.

A fucking terrible tragedy.

Paul had never heard his mother say *Fucking* and when added to *terrible tragedy* to become *fucking terrible tragedy*, it accurately summarized the afternoon and evening in August, 1955. *A fucking terrible tragedy.*

Paul concluded he was responsible. Richie was a victim of sexual abuse, because Paul failed to exercise good judgment, failed to protect his vulnerable friend, failed to say, *Don't go. I shouldn't have let him get in that car. There was something wrong with that guy. It was clear; he was dangerous. I knew it and I didn't do anything. Richie was torn. He wasn't sure he should go. He was waiting for me, his friend, to protect him. He was waiting for me, and I did nothing. And later, when his Mom called, I had a chance to end it. Maybe he wasn't assaulted until later, and if I had told his Mom that he got in a car with a strange guy who was Richie's foster father, maybe he could have been rescued before damage was done. Shit. I did it. I'm as responsible as the pervert who assaulted my friend. What kind of a friend am I? I let him down. I failed at friendship. Shit.*

Paul couldn't shed the guilt. It festered. He wanted to share his story with someone, anyone, liberate himself from responsibility, let the truth set him free, but sharing, asking for help would have been confessing and Paul didn't want anyone to know that he was responsible for his friend's sexual assault. Shame silenced Paul and he suffered in silence.

Paul and Richie remained friends. They played baseball together, golfed together and double-dated when Paul purchased his first car. They graduated high school together, and Richie was the only graduate to whom Paul gave a card, congratulating him for his accomplishment.

Richie remained in Anoka after attending college in Iowa, and taught school at the Senior High School. Richie and Paul remained friends. A group from their class, Frank, Richie, Paul, Cliff and others, held modest class reunions once a month, since 1971. The boys, then men, then seniors, bowled, golfed, played tennis, went to the movies, went to the bar or out to eat monthly. On the third Friday of the month immediately before Paul was diagnosed with lung cancer, the older men met for their 528th reunion.

Not everyone attended every reunion. Sometimes it was just Paul and Frank, or Richie, Cliff and Frank or another combination. Only once in 44 years had the men failed to get together. In January, 2001, Frank was on the west coast taping a golf tournament, the first where he shouted *You're da man*, Richie was at a school speech contest where his team surprised the competition and won the championship, Cliff and the others were in Florida, Texas or Arizona, so on the third Friday of January, 2001, Paul had a beer by himself and toasted the absent and missed his friends.

Every time Richie appeared, Paul quietly celebrated. Each time Richie did something that Paul believed was typical, normal, what other men typically did, Paul quietly celebrated. If Richie had a beer and said, *No more*, Paul celebrated. If he drank to drunkenness and slapped his friends on the back and slurred stories of their shared adolescence, Paul celebrated. If Richie missed a short putt and said, *Shit*, Paul celebrated. If a young woman in tight jeans walked by and Richie intently watched her pass, Paul celebrated. When Richie bought a truck, when he worked in dirt during the summers and sweated, when he purchased season tickets to Gopher hockey and when he stopped playing softball at age 54, because of arthritic knees, Paul celebrated and smiled.

Paul hadn't forgotten his role in a sexual assault, and as a lawyer, learned what victims of sexual assault carry with them for their lifetimes. Most are haunted. Many victims became abusers, perpetuating pain and devising it to the younger generation, some are depressed, some suicidal and others dysfunctional in nearly everything they do. When Richie smiled, Paul celebrated. When he worked year after year at the High School, and received awards for excellence, Paul celebrated. When Paul read the local newspaper's *Crime Report* or the jail roster and noted Richie's name was not on paper, he celebrated, a little. Richie's relatively normal life, didn't absolve Paul, but it lightened his load, knowing Richie wasn't an offender, mental health patient or victim of suicide.

Richie never married. He lived with another man, who taught at the Junior High School, but Paul didn't suspect homosexuality. They had separate bedrooms and Paul had oftentimes knocked on Richie's front door, unannounced and never discovered anything remotely suggesting anything other than a platonic relationship. Cliff believed Richie was gay, but after Cliff's recent revelation, Paul questioned his objectivity. *It's not just me.*

Richie was a complicated man with a complicated past. Paul was part of that past and, by omission, an unwillingness or inability to act, had contributed to the complications.

Fit, gray, clean-shaven, six feet tall, blue eyed, with a mouth full of white teeth, Richie looked wonderful for a 75 year old man. He walked to the foot of Paul's bed, stopped, smiled and asked, "How's my first Anoka friend?"

"God. You should've been in the movies. You look like the guy who travels to Italy alone and leaves with Sophia Loren."

"Thanks Paul. I almost feel guilty to say, I feel pretty good."

"Don't feel guilty about that. I suffer for habits indulged for more than a half-century. If I had said *No* to the first cigarette as you did, maybe we'd both be in Italy. Me with Mary, you looking for Sophia Loren."

"I remember your first cigarette. In the parking lot behind Dr. Rock's office on Jackson. A Camel. You stole three from your dad and wanted to share the experience with Cliff and me. Cliff said *Yes* and I said *No*. I was lucky. I don't remember why I declined. Probably just chicken. But, I don't remember ever getting together with you thereafter, when you didn't smoke."

Paul coughed. The cough was either the natural reaction to cancer in his lungs or manufactured to confirm what Richie implied.

"Tough habit. They had me at *Hello*. I tried to quit so many times. I knew what they were doing to me. I coughed every morning, sucked air every time I walked across a parking lot and caught every cold that set its sights on Minnesota and had a hell of a time ridding myself of the virus. Shit, I knew."

"I've heard."

"For nearly 20 years, I'd crush my pack of cigarettes each night before going to bed, destroying every cigarette in the pack, so that the next morning when I woke, I wouldn't have a cigarette to light. And every morning for 20 years, I woke, salvaged broken cigarettes in a crushed pack and smoked. If I 'd been appropriately aggressive, if I couldn't reconstruct a crushed cigarette, I'd fill a pipe bowl with tobacco from a crippled Camel and smoke it. Acupuncture, hypnosis, Nicorette gum, Quit Smoking Classes sponsored by the American Lung Association. I tried them all. Wasn't successful until the doctor said, *Paul, you have lung cancer and will likely be dead in six months*. Then, it was easy. Didn't have to crush a pack or chew nicotine gum. It was easy. Haven't had a cigarette in nearly a year and don't miss them at all. Wish there had been a less consequential reason to quit earlier, but here I am, at home, in hospice, a non-smoker."

"No room for guilt, buddy. We did what we did. No regrets. Life happened as it was supposed to happen. Don't punish yourself."

Paul wondered if Richie's words were an invitation. *No room for guilt? No regrets? Does he want me to ask? Does he want to talk about the summer before eighth grade? Does he want to share? Does he want to forgive me before I go?*

Uncertain, Paul ignored the elephant that had been in the room 62 years. "You're right. Cancer's plenty punishment."

After asking for and receiving permission, Richie sat in the chair that stood next to Paul's bed. He surveyed the room, saw the blonde box on the dresser and asked Paul if it was okay for him to look. He walked to the box, read the label and asked, "Frank? What is that?"

"It's Frank, or what's left of him. He died in his car across the street Tuesday. He didn't have family, so I have Frank."

Richie returned to the chair, sat quick and hard, slapped the arm-rests and showed as much emotion as Paul had seen from him in 64 years. "Damn. I didn't know. I saw him a few days ago. He told me he had a recording of Ernie Els he wanted to share with me. I told him to call. Frank always called, almost right away, so I wondered, but didn't think this. Wow! I had no idea."

"Yeah. He was here. We talked. He left, walked across the street and died. He thought he was telling me *Goodbye*. Little did I know, I was telling him *Goodbye*."

Richie washed his face with the palms of his hands, took a deep breath and summarized the consequence of age. "Our group is shrinking, Paul. Cliff, me and a couple of guys from the west side of town, Bruce and Lee, that's it. Two are in Florida full-time and two more live in an assisted living high-rise and can-not drive or walk to rendezvous, and if they did, they wouldn't remember why they were there or who we were. The rest, dead. Used to be 12 to 15 of us and now, when everyone shows, it's four. Five if you make it out of bed."

"Four. Don't count on five."

"We are fossils, my friend. We don't need doctors, we need archeologists."

 The old friends shared silence. Richie didn't speak, Paul didn't speak, nor did Frank.

"So, what do your doctors say, Paul? Any chance for recovery?"

"No. No recovery. This is hospice, palliative care. Not fighting the cancer, have accepted it will kill me. This is the home stretch at home. It's just a matter of time. I don't even see doctors anymore. There's nothing more they can do. I'm medically incorrigible. If I have trouble with pain, my nurse calls the doctors and they change the dosage of the pain meds and I float for a while, but that's it."

"I'm sorry Paul. You had a good run."

"Yup, I did. And even though I'm on my way out, it's not too bad. I sleep, I talk to family and friends, reliving good times and wait to learn what nobody here knows, what's on the other side?"

"You said *Nobody here knows*. I beg to differ." Richie looked at the dresser and winked. "Frank knows."

"But, he ain't sharing."

Richie laughed, but the laugh was short. He cleared his throat and taunted a 62 year old elephant. "You know Paul, it wasn't your fault."

Paul had made many mistakes in the 64 years since he met Richie and there had been consequences suffered by both as a result of those errors, but Paul knew exactly to what Richie referred. It was the mistake that had haunted Paul for decades.

"When I left the hospital, you never asked. I knew why. For years, I watched you turn white when I said I didn't feel well. I knew why. All those times you tried to set me up with friends of Mary, I knew why. You wondered, you suffered, but never asked. I should have told you, should have absolved you, told you it wasn't your fault, but I couldn't. I tried, but couldn't talk about that day. That day has haunted us both, but it should have only haunted me. I am the victim and you couldn't have prevented it. It wasn't your fault."

"But, I could have stopped you. I could have told your mom where you were. I could've stopped it, but didn't. I should've, but didn't. I'm responsible. At least in part."

Richie stood and gripped the bed-rails. He wiped a tear from his cheek and relieved Paul of responsibility. "You couldn't have changed things. It didn't matter what you would have said or done. I'd have gone anyway. It wasn't your fault."

"But...."

"But nothing, Paul. I knew what was going to happen. It happened before, when I was younger. I knew what he was going to do. I knew that my foster brother had been removed from his home and that he had been in prison. He repeatedly abused me as an eight year old and knew he would abuse me as a 13 year old.

Maybe a piece of me wanted to be abused. I don't know. It's all so sick. I don't know. But, what I do know is, you couldn't have prevented what happened. If it hadn't been that day, it'd have been another. We were on a collision course and nothing you could have done would have changed that."

"Why didn't you tell me?"

"I should have. I knew you felt responsible. But, telling the truth was almost impossible to do. I went with him knowing he'd abuse me. How could I tell you that? I'd be admitting I wanted it, that I was as sick as he was. I couldn't tell you that."

"But, you were a kid."

"No, Paul, I wasn't. I was a teenager. I knew better. I knew what would happen and I let it happen. Maybe I wanted it to happen. I was not only abused, maybe, I was willingly abused. In essence, I asked for it."

Paul pleaded for forgiveness, not the forgiveness he'd sought for 62 years, absolution for failing to protect his friend; instead, he sought forgiveness from the victim, for the victim. He wanted Richie to know that he wasn't responsible, couldn't have been. He wanted Richie to forgive himself, to know that he wasn't sick, but rather vulnerable prey for a perverted hunter. "But, Richie, in spite of what you say, you were a kid. Ten foster homes. Hopes raised, dashed. You were a kid. It wasn't your fault. You didn't ask for it, he took it from you."

Richie wiped tears from his face. "That's what I tell myself even 62 years later. It's what my therapists say. It's what authors of books say. Everyone says it, but, it's hard to rely on immaturity and imperfections or the influence of others. It was my decision. I try to remember I was young, scarred by a foster care system unable to find me a permanent home or protect me from predators or the whims of foster parents. Hell, in my sixth home, the foster parents sat me down, told me they understood I needed permanency and that they were willing to provide it, but six weeks later, they decided to take a road trip to California, so called Social Services and said, *We're going and he can't come with.* I was moved to number seven. I try to remember I was a kid and vulnerable, and most of the time, I get it, but it's tough."

Paul placed his bony, vein laden right hand on Richie's tanned left hand and let it draw pain from his friend. After five minutes of silence, punctuated with tears, Paul lifted his hand from Richie's, looked at the dresser and said, "What do you think, Frank? Have we fixed all that's wrong with the world?"

The men talked about the baseball championship, about Richie's home run, about Mrs. Ottenstroer, Mrs. Leonard and the Washington School playground. Richie explained that number ten, the home provided by the Richmonds, was nearly perfect, and although it took time, he learned to love his parents unconditionally. *Once a month, I place flowers at their gravesite and thank them for making me their son.*

"And I remember the first day of sixth grade. I was alone. I hoped to become part of something, but I was uncertain. It had been hard. I'd tried in the past, but it never worked. I was alone, but hopeful. And then a kid asked me if I played baseball and when I said *Yes*, he said, *You're on my team*." Richie took Paul's hands in his and said, "I'm still on your team. Thank you, my friend."

chapter twenty one

Paul took a bath after Richie left. He didn't leave his bed or clean himself, he laid there, just laid there and let Belle mop his shriveling body with a sponge and warm water. It felt good, refreshing. It took longer than it did weeks ago. Less muscle, less fat, more folds created seams that required scrubbing or the dirt that found hiding places would remain until the crematorium burned them away. Paul was dirty. Warm weather, drugs and immobility added to the accumulation of dead skin and dried sweat. Belle dumped and refilled her bucket twice and the last time she returned with clean, warm water, she washed Paul's face and hair. After she dried Paul with a fluffy white towel she found in the bathroom, Paul gave her directions. "Before my hair dries, please comb it and make sure that strand that likes to fall to my forehead, is where it should be, on the top of my head."

Belle did as she was instructed, and after dressing Paul with clean pajamas, handed him a hand-mirror and asked, "Well, what do you think?"

Paul held the mirror in front of his face. *Is that me? No, can't be. Too old, too gray, too thin, too moribund.* He looked for the boy who fell in love with Alice, the man who fell in love with Lisa, the boy who asked Richie to play baseball, the man who told Mary *I do* and did, for nearly fifty years, but he had a hard time finding him. There was a bit of that younger, healthier man in his tired eyes, and the lips that mouthed *I do, I love you, You're on my team*, hadn't changed much, except they drooped more toward his chin than they had in better days and were shadowed by slopes created by deep crevices that fell from each side of his nose to each corner of his mouth. He laid the mirror in his lap, smiled at what he remembered and what remained and asked, "Is this a trick mirror? It reveals an old man, not me. Must be black magic."

But, he felt clean, refreshed and that damn stubborn strand rested on the top of his head, not his forehead. "You do good work, Belle. Thanks."

Paul was a bit surprised at how much energy he burned, just lying there, getting a bath. He was tired. No marathon, no five-set tennis match or climb up the side of Everest, yet he was tired. He had a bath and was tired. He had just laid there, just lifted an arm, just let gravity and Belle roll him, and was tired, very tired. Drawn to sleep, but not knowing how many waking hours were left, or whether he would wake at all, Paul pried his eyes open with resolve, but ten minutes after he handed Belle the mirror, he closed his eyes and slept.

When he opened his eyes, Frank was dancing on the box that previously housed him. He was snapping his fingers and humming a song that was like, but wasn't, *Bohemian Rhapsody.*

When Paul felt his own fingers snap to the rhythm of the Freddy Mercury song, he pulled his hands from under the sheet and discovered they were covered with bugs, big bugs, small bugs, skinny bugs and fat bugs. He tried to rid his hands of the bugs by shaking his hands violently, but the bugs weren't dislodged when his hands shook, they dug in and multiplied. Paul called to Frank for help, but by the time his words crossed the room and landed on the blonde box, Frank was inside and the man who did a soft-shoe on the box lid, was the chinless, hairless, big bellied man who took Richie from the side of the road to a room filled with horror. Paul began shouting *Don't go, don't go*, but the perverted dancing foster father just grinned a prurient grin and laughed so loudly, Paul thought his ear drums would burst. Paul tried to protect his ear drums from the piercing laughter by inserting his fingers into his ears, but when he did, long, thin, bugs escaped from the tips of his index fingers and crawled into his ears where they waited for an order directing them to pierce the damaged ear drums. Paul began screaming for his mother and Jesus, begging them to help him escape and when he did, he heard a soft, reassuring voice from a place far away. The louder Paul screamed, the louder the reassuring voice called to him. *Paul. Paul. Paul. Paul.*

When Paul felt a large bug, the size of his hand, crawl on his shoulder, he opened his eyes more widely and discovered they hadn't been open at all. Belle was the source of the reassuring voice and the large bug was not a bug at all, but rather Belle's hand squeezing Paul's shoulder in an attempt to wake him and remove him from his hallucinogenic nightmare.

Paul looked at the box. It was closed. No one danced on its lid. He looked at his hands. Bug free. He took a deep breath, batted his eye lids, cleared his throat and looked again. No dead dancer, no bugs. He looked at his rescuer and thanked her for the parachute. "Thanks, Belle. That was quite a nightmare."

"Probably the meds. They tend to do that sometimes."

"I hope so. If that's what I'm in for when my heart stops beating and my brain waves no longer register, I'd prefer nothingness."

"It's the drugs, Paul. Don't fret the hereafter. It's wonderful."

Paul wanted to believe Belle. She was kind hearted and honest. She wouldn't lie, didn't have the chops for it. She believed what she said, but 15,000 miles away, a man wearing a khimar, leaned over to provide comfort to a fallen fellow jihadist, dying because an extremist Muslim detonated a suicide bomb a bit too close. Shrapnel entered the fallen man's body while body parts decorated his khimar. His friend, his fellow warrior and terrorist, looked to Mecca and said, *Don't worry, Allah will reward you for your actions, in the hereafter. It's wonderful.*

Can they both be right? Is Allah the only way? Is Jesus the only way? Are they mutually exclusive deities or friends providing different paths to the same wonderful hereafter? Paul didn't know the answer, had suspicions, but wasn't sure, but knew he'd know soon enough.

"Hope you're right, Belle. Can we do anything about the drugs if they give me that kind of nightmare?"

"I'll talk to your doctor, but if my recollection is right, it's the first time it happened to you, and if I'm right, it'll likely not happen again."

"I hope not. I don't like bugs."

As Paul brushed an imaginary bug from his right forearm and erroneously felt something crawl into his ear, Mary walked into the room with a card in hand. As she handed the card to Paul, she said, "Here. It's from Dot Haas."

"Why didn't she stop and say *Hello*?"

"Probably still too tough."

Paul opened the card and read. *So sorry to hear that things did not progress as you had wished. Sometimes, in spite of best intentions and Herculean efforts, they just don't. You were a good friend to Dave. He spoke kindly and warmly of you. I know you missed him. But, soon you may have an opportunity to renew your special friendship. For your sake, for Dave's sake, I hope so. When you see him, tell him I miss him and love him. Peace, Dot.*

Dave Haas. Law School classmate, roommate and Paul's best friend for the three most fun years of Paul's life, the years they attended Law School. Dave Haas, a confidant and source of comfort for nearly 50 years.

Paul attended law school at the University of North Dakota. He graduated from college with a degree in Political Science, scanned the want ads for jobs that required a degree in Political Science, found none, and applied to law school in North Dakota. The tuition was cheap, it was within a day's drive of home and was, at the time, the smallest law school in the United States.

Close, affordable, intimate. Perfect. If Paul had looked at a map to locate Grand Forks, home of North Dakota's law school, or if he had studied weather maps, he may have considered Iowa or Wisconsin, but he didn't, and applied to UND School of Law. He was accepted.

In the sixties, first year law students were required to attend an orientation on the Monday before classes began. At the orientation, a string of speakers gave the newbies information about law school and North Dakota. When the last speaker concluded with, *We're not the end of the world, but you can see it from here,* the new law students were given an opportunity to meet their classmates. Paul, intimidated by his classmates, believing only the best and brightest were accepted into law school and believing his admission was an error, that he didn't belong, was reluctant to meet his classmates and disclose his unworthiness with a modest vocabulary and imperfect grammar, so when orientation lectures ended and students began mixing, he slipped out a back door to smoke a cigarette and mine confidence.

As Paul lifted a flame to the Camel resting between his lips, he heard someone say, "Hey."

After bringing the flame to the cigarette and drawing smoke into his lungs, Paul turned to see who had greeted him with *Hey.* He was taller and heavier than Paul, yet not overweight or long enough to play center for a high school team. His hair was curly and sand colored, his eyes set deep and blue. Some of the students who remained in the law school building to chat, wore suits and ties and wing-tip shoes. Not him, not *Hey.* He wore blue jeans, a sweat-shirt and tennis shoes with a hole, that revealed a small toe, uncovered by a sock. He offered a calloused hand and said, "Dave Haas."

Paul shook his hand, introduced himself and offered Dave a Camel. "No thanks. I don't smoke, but I admit, it seems like everyone I know, smokes. Maybe I should start."

"Are you a first-year student?"

"I am. At least that's what the letter said. Maybe a mistake, but I guess I can attend classes."

Can attend classes. *Admission a mistake?* Dave wasn't perfect, made grammatical errors and didn't think he belonged. In less than ten-seconds, Paul determined he was like Dave, that they both belonged.

Relieved of pressure, Paul smiled. "Yeah. I have that same feeling. That I shouldn't be here, that I don't deserve to be here, that I don't belong. I look at all of those suits in there and think, *Wow, that's how they attend school in North Dakota?* But, my guess is, they all have those same insecurities."

"Probably. But, their advantage is, most went to undergraduate school here, so they know each other and their place amongst themselves. They've competed with one another and know they can succeed."

"Looks like they all went to the same store to buy their suits too."

"Probably wore them for graduation here last spring."

299

Paul had an ally, someone without a suit, someone who like him, hadn't attended classes with the people who mingled in the law school, someone who acknowledged misgivings and uttered grammatical errors. An ally, a fellow traveler, an admitted interloper.

Dave hitched his pants, cleared his throat and spoke. "Where are you from?"

"Anoka, just north of Minneapolis. You?"

"Mayville. Just south of here. My parents have a farm." He framed his tattered jeans and sweatshirt with his palms, and added, "No suit, just farm clothes."

Paul smiled. He wasn't from a farm, but he wasn't from the Board Room or a corporate office either. His clothes, khaki pants, a frumpy blue sweater and tennis shoes, like Dave's clothes, reflected his station in life. "I don't own one either. My last suit was bought for my Grandfather's funeral, sixteen years ago in 1948. If I could find it, it wouldn't fit."

When Paul finished his *Camel* and ended its life under his foot, he looked at his newfound friend, his ally, and said, "Well, should we meet our classmates?"

"Why not?"

As they walked to the back door they both had used to escape, Paul pulled at the waistband of his pants so that the zipper line was centered between his hips and smoothed wrinkles in his sweater with sweaty palms, while Dave stomped farm mud off his tennis shoes. Paul held the door open for Dave, who walked in, and as he did, said, "Fuck 'em."

They were surprised. In spite of their clothing, the other law students were down to earth, friendly, humble and interested in creating new friends. Some had shrill voices, others spoke with a baritone made for radio. The tallest student was a former college basketball player and the shortest, one of only two women in the class. Twenty were from Minnesota, one from Iowa, two from South Dakota, one very tan man was from California and the other 51 were from North Dakota. All were white. Most were in their very early twenties, having graduated from college the spring before, but five were older, veterans of the military and Vietnam. One was a retired general, a fifty-two year old native North Dakotan, who had served in World War II, Korea and Vietnam and was as frightened of law school as were Dave, Paul and the students dressed in suits.

During discussions with other first year law students, Paul and Dave learned that there would be a picnic sponsored by professional fraternities, for law students later that afternoon. Dave's rural eyes grew brighter and through upturned lips said, "Maybe this law school stuff will be fun."

They drove to the picnic together, sat at the same table, and when one met a new friend, the other did as well. The crowd was loud and by 4:00, rowdy. Everyone present drank beer dispensed from kegs which chilled in large metal buckets filled with crushed ice. When Paul returned from the keg with two glasses of beer, one for him and one for Dave, he articulated an observation. Free beer addled his brain and slurred his words, but Dave was also drunk, so he had no trouble interpreting what his new fried friend asked. "Why is it none of the guys we met this morning are here? Everybody here is a second or third-year student. Nobody from our class is here. I wonder why."

When introduced to the Student Bar Association President, a tipsy third-year student who wore shorts and a sweatshirt, Paul asked the more experienced student the question he had rhetorically posed to Dave and was told, "They're all home studying. Assignments for the first-year students are posted outside the Dean's Office. When classes start tomorrow, you're expected to be prepared. A professor will stand before a podium and ask first-year students questions about the day's assignments, ten seconds after class begins. No introduction. The clock strikes 8:00 and it starts. And the scary part is, these teachers feast on fear. They want everyone in that class to know that it is almost unforgivable to appear unprepared. So, they'll try to embarrass someone on the first day, so that everyone will walk into class frightened every day thereafter. Their goal is fear."

Too drunk to drive, Paul and Dave walked a crooked mile to campus, found the Dean's Office, wrote down their assignments and traveled to their respective homes, to study.

For Contracts, students were to read *The Death of Contract* and be prepared to discuss it in class.

Sober, Paul would have failed. Drunk, he had a hard time finding the first page. He tried to read. *Promissory estoppel. Plaintiff. Respondent. Petitioner. Appellee. Appellant. Legal consideration. Adequate consideration. Stare Decisis. Affirmed. Reversed and Remanded, with instructions. Llewellyn. Unconscionable. **Fuck**.*

He read the 30 page book twice. What he was unable to under-stand during his first reading, he was unable to understand during his second. He didn't know the words used and after he looked them up and wrote down the definitions, he forgot what he read in the dictionary when he returned to the text. The vowels and consonants were in the right places, the words were clearly En-glish words, but Paul had never before read them, spoken them or understood them. Drunk, he felt as if he were preparing for a class by reading lectures written in Swahili.

Paul surrendered to *The Death of Contract*, recognizing the pun-ishment for both him and contract, might be death, and opened his *Constitutional Law* text and read *Marbury v. Madison* as re-quired. As alcohol left his body, the letters were less fuzzy, the words not so. *If Appellant prevailed, does that mean the United States lost and the Supreme Court's powers were established or does it mean the Constitution is so confusing that the Supreme Court is required to interpret it?* **Fuck**.

Real Property. The difference between the present gift of a future interest and the future gift of a present interest? **Fuck.**

Dave and Paul sat in the large classroom next to one another at 7:55, and expressed mutual confusion. "I have no idea what I read. I tried, but couldn't understand." Both had headaches and upset stomachs, conceived by alcohol and born of anxiety. They, along with all of the other students in their class, sat quietly, nervously, awaiting the slaughter.

At 10 seconds before 8:00, Professor Richard Lord, who pre-ferred R. Lord, walked into the room, opened his booked, scanned a list of names and 20 seconds after walking in the room, at 10 seconds after 8:00, looked into the crowd of pale faces and said, "Mr. Toyle, is contract dead?" Mr. Toyle, wearing a sport-coat, white shirt and tie, crew-cut and red cheeks, had no idea what a contract was, let alone whether it was dead, but because he survived an hour of questions and answers, some pointed, some clearly designed to make him look stupid, he became a local folk-hero. After class, fellow students slapped him on the back, shook his hand and congratulated him for survival. Shell-shocked, Toyle smiled meekly, and like the others, apprehensively shuffled down the hall, on the way to *Real Property*.

Toyle was more-lucky in *Property*. Mr. Anderson, who looked like Elvis, but sounded like Brenda Lee, danced for an hour with Professor Bott, but in spite of the Professor's lead, was unable to distinguish between a present gift of a future interest and a future gift of a present interest.

Sally Jeffers, one of only two women in the class, an ex-para-legal, was asked by Professor Froilland, the *Constitutional Law* Professor, to explain *Marbury v. Madison*, and she was impressively able to do so, but, when she completed her explanation, Froilland scoffed and said, "If that's all there is to it, I better change jobs, for there's not much to teach. Miss Jeffers, get beyond the surface, ask important questions, don't be lazy and simply regurgitate the words. The law is about understanding what's behind the words. Anyone, even you Miss Jeffers, can recite what's written, but a good lawyer or good law student is expected to understand the words and analyze and apply them. Sophomoric effort, Miss Jeffers."

At 3:00 p.m., classes for the first day ended. All first-year students were intimidated. Goal accomplished; every one-L left class with sweaty palms, shaky fingers and cotton-mouth. Jeffers withdrew from law school that day and during the first week of classes, eight students who wore suits the day before classes began, decided law wasn't their calling.

Dave and Paul broke leases on separate apartments each had rented in Grand Forks, and moved into a small-house two blocks from campus, owned by Dave's brother. They found two-other first-year law students in need of good, cheap housing near campus, and invited them to join the former farmer and dishwasher. They did.

Dave and Paul studied together, drank alcohol together and chased undergraduate coeds together. Dave had been married and divorced before applying to law school. The divorce was her idea and Dave pined for his former lover. He enjoyed the attempts at repairing the hole in his heart drilled by his old girl with a new girl, but almost always, rejected the cure and continued to mourn. "I don't get it. It was perfect. Why? I just don't understand."

Twenty-one and unworldly, Paul had no answers. When it got tough, academically or emotionally, Paul put a flame to a Camel and said, "Let's get a beer." And they did.

During spring breaks of their second and third years of law school, they travelled to Florida together and during the summer between first and second–year they drove to western Montana and camped in the mountains. After graduation, Paul and Dave drove to California, where they toured Hollywood's Television City and attended an Elvis Presley concert.

Paul sat for the bar examination in Minnesota and Dave in North Dakota. After each passed the bar, Paul received a *Greetings* letter from the U.S. Army and Dave found work with the North Dakota Insurance Commissioner. When Paul survived Basic Training and Vietnam, he returned to Anoka and began to practice law. The two law school friends stayed in touch, by letter and telephone and in June, 1967, after Paul was discharged from active duty, he answered a knock on his door and discovered it had been rapped by Dave.

"I'm selling cars in St. Cloud. Thought I'd stop and see my old friend."

Surprised, recognizing that a law degree wasn't required to sell Fords, knowing that Dave had a good law job in Bismarck and had forfeited it for car sales, Paul asked, "What the Hell, Dave? We suffered for three years. For what?"

"I decided to end the suffering at five years. Three years of law school followed by two years of lawyering made it clear. I'm no lawyer. It never fit. I'm more comfortable in blue jeans than a three-piece suit. I should've followed Jeffers out the door. But, it was fun. I have no regrets, but if I stayed, knowing what I know, knowing what I feel, I would've created regrets. It was time to end the masquerade."

A Chevrolet man, Paul bought seven Fords from Dave. Dave met Dot when he sold her a 1968 Ford Fairlane and proposed to her when she upgraded to a 1969 Galaxy. Paul was Dave's best man, and when Paul married Mary, Dave was the groomsman who stood next to Cliff, Paul's best man.

Dave lived in St. Cloud, and Paul in Anoka. They lived 48 miles apart, an hour's drive, but saw each other only sporadically, likely four or five times a year. When something important stamped itself on a life, when a child was born, when a doctor's diagnosis was unkind, when children celebrated a big win or survived a close call, when one of the two felt vulnerable and needed someone who knew and cared, they bridged the short gap that separated them, and met. Paul loved and relied on Dave and Dave relied on and loved Paul.

At 10:30 p.m., on July Fourth, 2014, Paul received a telephone call, which his cell phone identified as placed by Dave. Paul smiled, tapped the button that said *Accept* and spoke into his phone. "David. How are you, my friend?"

After ten seconds of silence, Paul heard a voice, but it wasn't Dave's, instead it was Dot's. "Dave's dead, Paul. I'll fill you in tomorrow."

One month short of the fiftieth anniversary of their introduction, Dave's voice became silent and Paul could no longer rely on his friend for comfort, insight or a new car. He helped carry Dave's box from a hearse into a church in Mayville and delivered the eulogy.

I've known many longer than I knew Dave Haas. There are those I saw more often than I saw Dave Haas. I've known others longer and seen others more frequently than I saw Dave, but with the exception of my wife, children and parents, there is no relationship that I have had, that has been more important to me, than my relationship with Dave Haas. If I needed a dollar, Dave was there. If I needed direction, Dave was there. When I struggled, when happiness was fleeting or gone, Dave was first person I called, and with him, I found happiness and peace.

He was a famer from here in Mayville, but he was much more than that. He was a father, who loved his children and raised them as happy kids. He was a devoted husband to Dot, who filled a hole in his heart and helped him fly without wings for nearly a half century. He was a solid member of this community and the community he called home for the last 45 years, volunteering to satisfy needs and donating time and money to alleviate pain and suffering. And he was my friend. I miss him now. My heart is breaking and for the first time in 50 years, Dave can't take my call, meet me, or comfort me.

As tears fell to the paper that Paul brought to the pulpit, he stopped, walked to the long blonde box that held his friend, tapped it twice, returned to the lectern and said, *Goodbye my friend. Until we meet again.,*

Paul read what Dot wrote again. *But, soon you may have an opportunity to renew your special friendship. For your sake, for Dave's sake, I hope so. When you see him, tell him I miss him and love him. Peace, Dot.*

Paul wiped a tear from his cheek and concluded death offered opportunities not available to the living. Anticipating an opportunity to hug his old, dear friend, Paul called out to Mary, "Tell Dot, I will do just that."

Paul pulled the pen from under his disappearing ass and grabbed the paper from the table and wrote.

Dear Dave:

It's been more than a year since I heard your soft, assuring voice, 13- months since my rudder was plucked from the water that is drowning me. When a Doctor told me, treatment was ineffective and that I should accept my fate and prepare to die, I reached for my phone, to call you. I had questions, fears and mottled solutions that nagged me and I needed guidance. You had always provided that guidance, but when my fingers activated my phone and tried to reach you, I remembered, you couldn't be reached, at least not by telephone. For half a century, I relied on you and when I needed you most, you weren't there. Not your fault; I understand; I'll be unavailable soon as well.

There's good and bad news.

The bad. My last breath will be taken soon. My joints will stiffen and my fluids will accumulate as gravity demands, unfettered by circulation. If my kids, grandkids or wife need my advice, comfort or just a hug, I won't be able to give it. I will be indisposed. The bad news is, I'll be dead and unavailable to the living.

The good. I never met Lincoln or had an opportunity to thank my dad's best friend for saving his life, by stepping in front of a bullet intent on killing my dad and erasing me. I always wanted to know if Adam was happy with Eve or wanted options and why Lyndon Johnson, an otherwise caring, sensitive man, sent boys to die in a war he knew he couldn't win. I haven't had a chance to talk to you for 13 months and share my secrets and fears, or collect your advice and wisdom. Soon, I will meet Abraham Lincoln, thank Harold Blair, discuss war with LBJ and the beginning with Adam, and most importantly, talk to you. The good news is, I'll be dead and available to the dead.

So, my friend, get ready. I'm coming and will be bringing someone with me. I'll need someone to show me the lay of the land, and if necessary, to lobby for my inclusion into that part that's warm, comfortable, wonderful. If you know Harry Blair, Lincoln, LBJ or Adam, or see my mom and dad, please tell them, I'm on my way.

Sincerely,

Paul.

P.S. Is it true that the sins of the father fall on the son? If so, that's really unfair to Randy. He didn't know. And as I ask that question, I must say, I don't know what my Dad did behind closed doors. Maybe lobby first and then talk to Lincoln and LBJ. Thanks, my friend.

chapter twenty two

When a baby, fresh from his mother's womb, Paul slept 20 hours a day. When a teen with a growing body that zapped energy as it stretched and grew, he slept ten hours a day. When he attended college and law school and had classes early in the morning and beer late at night, he slept six hours a night and when he worked as a prosecutor, then public defender, then private practitioner, he tried to turn out the lights at 11:00 and was roused by the alarm clock at 7:00. When he was first diagnosed with cancer, anxiety made it hard to sleep, and he slept fitfully only five or six hours a night. After the doctors said, don't worry, it won't help, you'll be dead soon, no matter what you or we do, the anxiety disappeared and Paul was able to sleep eight to nine hours a night. When he first returned home to die, as his body failed and drugs delivered immunity from pain, he slept 12 hours a day. A week later, as his journey neared its destination, on the day he received a sponge bath and wrote a letter to his dead friend, he slept 16 hours and while awake, fought the urge to sleep for three hours, leaving him with only five hours each day unobstructed by sleep or the overwhelming desire to sleep.

At birth, Paul, like all other infants, relied on his mother for food, for warmth, for comfort, for everything. He was vulnerable and dependent, and without his mother, he would have died. He was weaned from his dependency on his mom and by the time he walked in rice fields in Vietnam, he was independent and able to care for himself without much assistance. And as he laid in a bed with side-rails, he understood his independence had vanished. He relied on others for warmth, for food, for medicine, for comfort, for everything.

As a baby, he cried. When he was hungry, he cried, when he was frightened, he cried, when he was dirty and in need of cleaning, he cried. He cried and cried and cried. As a healthy, younger man, tears never welled in his eyes, nor was he ever required to gasp for air in between sobs. But, on the day he was washed with a sponge, as he laid in bed, waiting to die, understanding *goodbye* meant **goodbye**, that he wouldn't see his grandchildren marry, his son retire or another Christmas or Fourth of July, he cried.

The end was like the beginning. Paul cried, needed to sleep 20 hours daily and relied on others to survive when he entered the world, and now, 75 years later, as he was leaving the world, tears often welled in his eyes, he snored and dreamed 20 hours a day and needed help to eat, to wash, to dress, to survive.

Separated by 75 years, the beginning was much like the end.

But 75 years ago, it was all before him, and now, it was all behind him. Then, he had a future, now, he had a past. He smiled. *It's mostly behind me, but I had a good life. Few regrets, many accomplishments. I did what I could and have left a pleasant im-print on others. I'll be gone, but I'll live on, in the memories of those I touched and the impact I had on others, which blossoms and grows long after I draw my last breath. It's been good.*

Paul closed lids wiped clean by Belle, batting tears from experienced eyes, and like a baby, slept. His sleep was without dreams, without pain, without angst. The slate was full, the smile broad and the legacy nearly complete.

When Paul opened his eyes, it was dark. He could see a crescent moon and a smattering of stars outside his shadeless window. A breeze that smelled of lakeshore in the summer wafted into the room and for a short moment, Paul thought he was 28 and in Spooner, at the cabin, near the water. He coughed up a string of phlegm, spit it into a Kleenex, remembered where he was and looked at the clock. It read 2:45. Still, dark, the middle of the night. He felt something against his right leg, flush and extending from his quad, across his knee and terminating at his calf. It moved. As he lifted his head from his pillow to determine what warmed his leg and smelled of lake cabin, the warmth lifted its head as well and flapped it large ears back and forth releasing small strands of brown and white fur into the air. Cosmo.

Cosmo was Paul's third last dog. Mary considered a dog, another mouth to feed, a child incapable of independence, a barking intruder, dog hair, a four-legged inconvenience that required someone to trek into the cold and rain when its bowels moved and an anchor to home when she wanted to stay out late or travel to warmer climates in the winter. Paul considered a dog, loyal, warm, loving and necessary.

313

When Paul and Mary met, Paul had a dog. When Mary and Paul began sleeping together, Beatle (the talent of four men in one dog) shared their bed and most often, chose to sleep next to Paul, on the side of the bed Mary occupied.

"Paul, get this dog out of our bed."

"It was his before yours."

"Are you suggesting he has as much right to this bed as me?"

"No. You're my wife; he's my dog. He walks on four, you're upright, on two. You wear shoes, he doesn't. He can't cook or bear children. If I have to choose, I'll choose you. Without an option, I'd send him to the floor."

"Well?"

"There are options. He'd be miserable on the floor. He's been sleeping on my bed for years. I let him sleep with me, before there was a you. It wouldn't be fair to him now. He's just a stupid dog; he wouldn't understand."

"*I* don't understand."

"When I plucked him from the box while his mother growled at me, I made a commitment, as I did when you and I stood on the altar. I can't break my vows, to you, or to him. It wouldn't be fair."

"When you plucked him from the box, did you tell him he'd be able to sleep in your bed, between you and your wife?"

"No. But I told him I'd give him a good home and do what I could to make him happy. He just wants to be close to us. Me and you. It makes him happy."

"Close to us? I don't think so."

"Before you and I shared a bed, he slept on my left, nearer the window. You climbed in, and he started sleeping to my right, so he could be close to both of us. It's not just me he wants. It's you too."

"He changed sides, so he could be between us. He has no interest in me, except to the extent he's interested in separating you and me."

"You give him too much credit. He's a dog. Not capable of such sophisticated reasoning." Paul reached across the bed, to caress Mary's shoulder and confirm that Beatle would not ever be an obstacle impeding love between a husband and wife, and when he did, Beatle lifted his big yellow head from the bed and bumped Paul's arm, moving his hand from Mary's shoulder. "See, he has no idea."

Mary didn't answer. She turned to her left side, facing the wall, not her husband. After an uncomfortable silence, a not-to-be-pregnant pause, Paul slapped the bed and looking at Beatle who stood after Paul slapped the bed, said, "Down."

When Beatle hit the floor and moaned his disapproval, Mary turned, faced her husband and said, "Thank you."

Beatle was two when Paul and Mary met. After three children filled the Thomas house with laughter and tears, Beatle, then 14, slowed and took the stairs, one at a time. The kids jumped on the old dog, poked him in the eye with blocks and dolls, pulled his fur and tail and slapped him when they wanted him to move. Beatle yawned, licked his paws and wagged his tail.

On a summer day in 1980, on her way to three playdates, Mary strapped the children in car seats, and backed her van from the garage. Two minutes after she left the house, she returned and called for Paul. "Paul, come here."

Beatle was under the wheels of Mary's van, unable to move, because after a tire rolled over him, a paw was pinched between the driveway and the front passenger tire of Mary's van. Paul reached for Beatle, and as he did, Beatle bit the hand that offered rescue. With a bloody hand, Paul removed Beatle's imprisoned paw from between the driveway and tire and pulled him from under the van. Beatle didn't move, but rather looked at Paul and closed his eyes, never to open them again.

Paul violated two city ordinances and a state law when he buried Beatle in his residential back yard. He didn't care and knew no one else would either.

Mary felt terrible.

Beatle was a good dog. The kids loved him and he tolerated them in warm and loving ways, gently and with a wagging tail. When kids cried, he sat at Mary's feet while she held and comforted sick or frightened children, looked at her with warm brown eyes, seemingly saying, *We're in this together*. He was comforting *and* easy. He only needed to be fed once a day and found his own way to the small strip of woods to do his duty, twice a day. He slept on their bed, but with some effort, learned to lay on the side of the bed between Paul and the wall. He rarely barked, never had in-house accidents and when things were hectic and his presence would have exacerbated chaos, he found a corner and laid quietly, waiting for the circus to end.

Mary felt, terrible.

"It was an accident. It's okay. I don't blame you."

A year after Beatle was buried in the backyard, when grass grew over him, hiding his grave, when time turned Mary's guilt into a fading, yet uncomfortable memory, Paul chided her. "Were you afraid that if I was required to choose, I would've chosen Beatle?"

Paul gave the kids a black cocker spaniel as a Christmas gift in 1982. When Kota bit Randy's face in 1984, Paul found Kota a new home. In 1985, Paul brought a Golden Retriever home and named him Beamer, after a character in the *Rockford Files*. Beamer was a good dog, with bad genes. He had epilepsy, a faulty hip and in 1992, quietly died on the kitchen floor.

Paul buried Beamer next to Beatle and when he put the shovel away, Mary stood on the garage apron and said, "No more."

After six months without a dog to greet him at the front door after an anxious day in court, after six months without a dog to sit at his feet when he smoked the last cigarette of the day, while children slept in their beds and Mary watched the news in their bedroom, Paul brushed his teeth, shed pants and a shirt for pajamas, crawled between sheets and said, "One more. I miss having a dog around."

Mary could have objected and wanted to object, but didn't.

Tundra was big, stubborn and yellow. He was kind, but stupid, and was devoted to Mary, in spite of her disinterest. He followed her. Everywhere she went, he went. If anyone wanted to know where Mary was, they needed to know where Tundra was, and if they were interested in locating Tundra, they simply needed to locate Mary. Before his sixth birthday, Tundra bolted from the backyard, attempting to catch Mary's car, and was killed by a moving van carrying furniture to the home of Paul's new neighbor, the assistant pastor of Paul's church.

Two months later, Paul said, "One more," and brought a seven-year-old lab mix home from the local shelter. Trax, another gentle and good dog, who was also devoted to Mary, lived to the old age of 15, before leaving Paul dogless yet again.

A year after Trax's death, *Mary* sat at the kitchen table and asked, "One more?"

Paul and Mary scanned the internet like two young kids looking for their first dog. They researched breeds and after they decided to buy a Springer Spaniel, researched breeders. They completed an application, stomached a home-study and brought Cosmo home.

Paul believed dogs adjusted, morphed, became what their owners wanted. Dogs Paul owned when he was young and active, were young and active, running with Paul, swimming with Paul and rising with Paul and the sun, signaling the new day with a wagging tail and wide-open eyes. Dogs Paul and Mary owned when they were parents of young children, were like the kids, playful, curious and challenging.

Cosmo was like Paul. His disposition was older, more mature and his interests, refined and quiet. He was a hunter who preferred to hunt squirrels, deer, chipmunks and rabbits, through a shadeless window, from the bed. He chased balls thrown down the hill, but returned them slowly, deliberately, and was partial to long walks on the end of a leash, walking beside Paul. At night, after Paul laid on the bed, Cosmo laid on the floor, at the foot of the bed, waiting. After Mary closed her eyes and mumbled in a dream, Paul whispered *Okay,* and Cosmo jumped to the bed and slept at Paul's feet.

Without children at home, while Mary busied herself with social work, technology and friends, Cosmo was Paul's constant companion. Paul rubbed his offered belly when he walked into the room and scratched behind his ears when Cosmo rested his head on Paul's lap. When C.O.P.D. and worn joints ended Paul's career as a runner, Cosmo and Paul stopped running and walked an hour each evening after supper.

When doctors told Paul, his lungs were corroded and filled with cancer, they suggested he limit his contact with animals, suggesting that animal dander and fur could compromise his lungs further and make it difficult to breath. While he treated, while he hoped for remission, a cure and a longer life, Paul limited his contact with Cosmo, but when doctors told him, it was over, that remission and cure were not possible and his long life would end at 75, Paul sat on the leather couch and asked Cosmo to put his head in his lap. When he did, Paul caressed his head and made both Cosmo and him happy.

And at 2:30 a.m., Cosmo rested comfortably at Paul's side, providing comfort. Paul scratched behind his friend's ears, closed his eyes and returned to sleep. He dreamed of confirmation, when what he dreaded was confirmed.

"Mr. Thomas, I'm Dr. Ford." Paul was oftentimes surprised by a doctor's appearance. They preach good health, a modest diet of greens and fruit, exercise and moderation, yet often look like fried chicken, scotch and a sedentary, frenetic life. Dr. Ford looked-liked he preached. He was long, thin, sinewy, pale, with a splash of sun and measured.

"Not so happy to meet you Dr. Ford, but I've been told you are very good at what you do." *If there is anything to be done.*

"Your doctor sent me his file. I've had a chance to look at it." He paused. He turned to the computer screen in the room and read. He scrawled through the electronic documents, read again and took a deep breath, looking for the appropriate words. He scratched the left side of his head with his left index finger, crossed his feet, uncrossed them, looked at his watch and then the screen again. He blinked his eyes two times, then closed them inviting darkness into the silence. His palpable discomfort was more articulate than words. He turned his stool on wheels to face Paul, slapped his knees and ended the silence while raising the stakes. "I've done this for many years, and it is always hard to deliver bad news. And the news is bad."

Doctors who preach, those who suggest changes in lifestyle to lengthen life and give it more pizzazz, those who recommend exercise, a diet flooded with fruits and vegetables, those who review charts and modestly shake their heads in disgust when reading about their patient's use of tobacco or overuse of alcohol, shouldn't be overweight with tans that suggest much too much time in the sun. Dr. Ford was unlike those medical contradictions, smug fat doctors who counseled a fat free diet or medical men alcoholics who drank until drunk each night, yet counseled moderation. He showed no disgust, nor did his appearance reflect a commitment to hedonism. With compassion and without words, he smiled sympathetically. Paul ended the silence. "It's not news, Doctor, I've figured it out. I'm neither stupid nor Pollyannaish"

The doctor cleared his throat. *Nerves? Maybe a smoker's throat? Nah.* "The masses revealed in your x-ray, appear to be cancerous tumors. They're large, numerous and appear in every lobe of each lung. At this point, surgery is not an option." He returned to the screen, but it was clear, it was only a preserver, a tool, an opportunity to think, plan and carefully choose words.

"Can anything be done?"

"There is a great deal that can be done. And will be done."

"And will it be effective?"

"Unknown. Lung cancer is tough. And yours appears to be advanced. Cure? Doubtful. Remission? Maybe. Chemotherapy and radiation can shrink the tumors so that surgery can remove them, but it's highly unlikely all of the cancer can be removed. And there is the possibility that cancer has metastasized to other organs. There are tools. We'll use them all. They will likely extend your life, but for how long it can be extended, is impossible to say at this time. We'll take it step-by-step, evaluate, re-evaluate and make necessary adjustments as your body suggests."

"The next step?"

"I'm going to schedule additional testing. A biopsy and body scans. We'll examine the tissue so that we know exactly with what we're dealing and find out if it's creeped beyond your lungs, to other organs. Once we know exactly what you have, we'll fashion a program designed to attack what's attacking you."

"Prognosis?"

"Too early to say. Guarded at best. There is a lot of dark in your lungs, but, medicine has made great progress and I'm hopeful we can help." Understanding Paul wanted more, recognizing hope fuels healing and hope can be a number, he looked at the screen, panning for honest words that might plant hope. "If you didn't celebrate Christmas, I'd be surprised and disappointed. If you celebrated your 85th birthday, I'd be surprised and I'd thank God and medicine. More than that, I just can't say now."

"Understood. I accept that it's not clear. You provided some hope and I'm not interested in false hopes. I appreciate it. Thanks."

"Wish I could say more. We'll figure it out."

"Thanks."

"Questions?"

"None. I'm sure I'll have them, but you've answered the ones I had coming in."

"Good. I'll send in Millie. She'll schedule the tests. If you have questions that nag at you, those that make it hard to sleep or smile, please call or ask on MyChart. Sometimes it'll take a while for me respond, but I will, and almost always on the day you ask. I'd rather be here an additional ten minutes each day addressing your fears than know you're living in misery because you have questions and they're not being answered."

"Thanks, Doctor. You may regret that invitation. I have lots of fears and am prolific with a keyboard."

"Not to worry. If I think it's getting out-of-hand, and I don't think it will get-out-of-hand, I'll let you know."

After an exchange of *Thank you's*, and a hand shake, Doctor Ford left Paul to contemplate the rest of his short life.

A fucking Rambler. A fucking Rambler. Immediately after break-in, begins to sputter and at 75,000 miles, dead. A Mercedes? 200,000 and running strong. BMW? Going on and on and on. Toyota, Subaru? Forever, damn near. Not me. A fucking Rambler. Rusted chassis, knocking engine, upholstery splitting at the seams because the stitching was faulty and the fabric cheap. Rattles, exhaust fumes in the passenger compartment, a radio that can't maintain a signal. A fucking Rambler. Fuck.

"Thank you, Millie."

Cosmo scratched behind an ear and transformed the bed with side-rails into a rubber raft on a churning sea. Shaken by his dream and his dog, Paul opened his eyes, and as he did, Cosmo relieved his itch and returned to sleep. Paul remembered every detail of his dream. It wasn't really a dream, but rather a recollection delivered while asleep. It was easy to remember, because it was all true, all accurate, all relived day after day, night after night.

Doctor Ford and Paul met online nearly daily and face to face nearly weekly for almost two years. Paul had done as Dr. Ford prescribed. Biopsy? Large cell carcinoma. Body scan? Metastasized to lymph nodes in the chest, and perhaps to bones. Radiation. Chemotherapy. Blood tests. Shrinking? Disappearing? Growing? Shrinking? Magically appearing in places not previously poisoned. Numbers up, numbers down. Too late, too early. Not yet.

Two years after they first met, Paul was scheduled to meet with Dr. Ford. He sat in a plastic chair in a small room waiting for the doctor to appear. He waited and waited. When the door opened, the man who darkened the door's frame, was not Dr. Ford. The man in white was twenty years younger than Ford, and light-skinned with teeth so white, it was clear he'd never smoked, consumed refined sugar or caffeine. He offered a hand and an explanation. "I'm Doctor Alms. Dr. Ford had a heart-attack. So, I'm taking over your case. If that's okay with you."

"Will he be all right?"

"Not sure. It just happened last night. I hope so. He's a good man."

"I'm very sorry to hear that. He's been very good to me. If you see him, please give him my best wishes."

"I will." Dr. Alms was unafraid of offense. He didn't choose his words, didn't formulate a speech, he simply spoke. He had looked at Paul's chart before he stepped into the examination room and had no need for crutches, so he looked at Paul and said, "Mr. Thomas, it looks like medicine has done all it can do. Your cancer is not giving up, and it's getting close to the finish line. Further treatments won't delay the end, they'll only cause you additional discomfort, so Dr. Ford had decided to tell you to abandon further treatment. I reviewed your chart quite closely and must reluctantly tell you, I agree with Dr. Ford. I'm sorry, but it does not appear that there is anything more to be done."

Fucking Rambler.

Doctor Ford didn't leave the hospital alive. In spite of fruits, vegetables, a lean body and a measured approach, he was cremated and buried. Paul attended his service and thanked his childless widow for the Doctor's care. "He was a good man who helped me immensely. I am so very sorry for your loss." *A Studebaker? Maybe. Certainly not a Toyota, Subaru, BMW or Mercedes. Fucking Studebaker.*

Cosmo's itch resurfaced and he scratched. Paul slapped the bed and after Cosmo looked, said, "Come here, boy." With larger digits and enough strength remaining to exorcise an itch, Paul scratched the creases between ears and skull and said, "You're a good boy. Certainly at least a Subaru."

Cosmo laid down and rested his back against Paul's side. When he was as close to Paul as he could get, Cosmo retracted his paws, dug them into the bed and extended his legs, pushing himself closer, sealing the bond between dog and master. He turned his big head to Paul, satisfied himself that he was where he wanted to be, dropped his liver-and-white covered crown to the bed and slept.

chapter twenty three

*W*hen Paul opened his eyes, it was either tomorrow or the day after tomorrow. He wasn't sure. The sun was above the horizon, lighting the sky and casting short shadows that laid east of their principals. *1:30?* Paul turned his head and looked at the clock with illuminated numbers, that rested on the bed-stand that stood sentry to the narrow window in his bedroom's south-east corner. *1:42. Not bad.*

Mary walked into the room, carrying her iPad, a dish-rag and her head high. She smiled. Her face was full of color, suggesting she had spent time in the sun while Paul slept. "Welcome back."

"Is it today or tomorrow? I can't tell if I slept 10 hours or 34."

"It's today. You slept through the night and into the day. I checked on you every hour since seven this morning, and every time I checked, you were sleeping. You weren't moving. Peaceful, that's how you looked. Your breathing was clear and measured and you were smiling, darn near smirking. It was a mischievous grin, the kind you flashed when we were young and the kids fell asleep. Not sure what could make you smile like that now, but it looked like you were enjoying yourself."

"You'll never know, because I don't know. It must've been good. I don't smile like that when I'm awake, because I don't have those thoughts anymore. I know my limitations. Maybe in dreams I can still do what I did when I was young." Paul flashed a mischievous grin. "Maybe you should leave so I can go to sleep."

"Depends. Who's in your bed while you're sleeping? If it's that floosy down the block, I think I'll bang pots and pans for a while, but if it's me, I'll be happy to leave you to your sleep and dreams."

"How could it be anyone else?"

Modestly embarrassed by Paul's warm words filled with prurient implications, blood rushed to Mary's sensitive cheeks, increasing the color produced by the sun, while color left Paul's face as he remembered and he regretted, that there had been someone else. Pallid, shame filled, Paul wondered if he should unburden himself by confessing to his transgressions, his dalliance, his love affair with a woman who had been dead almost 40 years. Mary, loyal, sacrificial, generous, unsuspecting and loving, didn't deserve what Paul gave in the early seventies. She kept his oldest child happy, healthy and fed, while keeping Paul's home warm and inviting and her passions for only Paul. Paul left Lisa's bed, her arms and her kisses and returned to Mary and Lauren, tired, guilty and uninterested in passion. He had divided his heart and the part that remained for his family, for Mary and Lauren, and later, Randy, was insufficient. And in spite of his weakness, his infidelity, Mary was always there for him when he returned from his bouts with deceit, with a kiss, an *I missed you*, innocent questions about his trip and enthusiasm about their future.

Mary had deserved better and Paul had failed her. While Mary waited and worried, Paul cheated. Paul's tryst with Lisa haunted him, hanging darkly in the sky between his home and the heavens. *A ceiling, a barricade? Will the haunting continue after my death?*

Paul couldn't do anything about what he had done. That was over, not fixable. He fucked up and would take his violations with him to his grave. He was an adulterer, then, always. No do-overs; it was done. He was what he was. That worried him.

Paul believed his afterlife would be influenced by the attitude and mood he carried to his death. He expected there would be a carryover, from life to death. The hereafter was not a new beginning uninfluenced by the life lived, but rather a continuation of that life into a vastly different spot, a spot defined, in part by Paul. If he died with a smile, happy and guilt-free, he would celebrate in the hereafter, however, if he died burdened and consumed by guilt, he could matriculate to a dark foreboding place.

He wondered if he would be punished forever for his blunder, his deceit and infidelity if he didn't confess and cleanse his soul. He suspected that if he confessed, he would be set free by revealing the truth, and the shame and guilt would evaporate and he would pass to eternal bliss, but knew the consequences would be great.

Embarrassed, blushing, Mary stood at the foot of her dying husband's bed and smiled. She didn't know and her ignorance was liberating and joyful. If Paul unburdened himself, if he confessed and saved his soul, if he told Mary she was wrong, that their life hadn't been blissful and pure as she believed, if he told her he was a cheat, an adulterer, he would destroy Mary's lifetime of happy memories, her belief in idyllic love, loyalty and commitment. Paul weighed the options. His eternity, Mary's earthbound happiness. Infinity or a few years? Forever or a fortnight?

The decision was evident, clear. He was wrong; he had made the mistake; he tarnished the relationship by succumbing to temptation and desire. It was his mistake and he'd suffer the consequences rather than hurt Mary.

Tempting the devil, but delivering Mary to the place she deserved, Paul said, "No one but you, Mary. Here and in my dreams, always only you."

Sensitive, quiet, demure, Mary blushed further. "That's what I thought."

Mary clasped Paul's left hand in her hands and in silence, thanked her God for her husband. She was lucky, blessed. *Thank you.* "Pastor James is here. She's sharing stories with the kids, but came to see you. It's up to you. She'd like to see you, but won't be angry or sad if you'd rather visit with the kids."

"Send her in. I've avoided her long enough. Maybe she can absolve me of my sins."

"What sins?"

Paul grinned, not quite mischievously, but not wholly innocently. "That's between God and me."

Mary smiled. "I'll send her in. Will the list of sins be long? Do you need more than a couple of hours?"

"Depends on how specific she wants me to be. In any event, not more than a couple of days."

As they both laughed, Mary innocently, Paul sheepishly and deceptively, Mary turned and walked from the room.

Sandy James walked into Paul's hospice, carrying a cup of coffee. The mug read, *Sundays are for Golf.* The 40 year old cup, taken from the Thomas cupboard and filled with coffee made in Paul's fifty year old percolator, was given to Paul on a Fathers' Day when the kids still lived with their parents. Sandy set the mug on the bedside table and shook Paul's weak and disappearing right hand. She smiled, retrieved her cup, and likely for the first time, read its message. Embarrassed by the mug's message, Paul apologized. "Sorry about that."

Sandy smiled. "It doesn't say *Sundays are Exclusively for golf.* I sometimes hit a golf ball on Sunday afternoons, after church. A good mix. No offense taken."

She was a fit 43 year old woman with short, dishwater-blonde hair and an unrelenting smile. She was a runner. Paul oftentimes saw her jogging around Anoka, near the golf course, downtown, on country roads and on the track near the high school, smiling. In the rain, the sun or under white cumulus clouds, she ran and she smiled. Lean, she carried no excess weight on her short torso and her long legs churned effortlessly as she ran and ran and ran. As she sipped coffee in a mug that read *Sundays are for Golf*, she wore a joggers' suit made of blue nylon, with a Nike swoosh over her left breast. As almost always, she was on her way to or from a run.

"No collar, no robes. I assume this visit is unofficial. That's probably a good sign."

"It's as official as you want it to be, Paul. I was in the neighborhood, just finished a run, and thought I'd stop by and see how you, Mary and the kids were doing. Always concerned about the flock."

"Thanks. I appreciate it, and I'm sure Mary and the kids do as well."

"Glad to be here."

"I've often thought that the ministry is a lot like lawyering. We have a lot in common. My profession is similar to yours."

The Pastor asked for clarification. "In what ways?"

"We typically deal with people who are in crisis. They're hurt or dead and they or their survivors call on us to help them through the difficult times. What they tell us is protected by confidentiality rules and we do what we can to relieve the pain."

"Interesting."

"I don't sing hymns or speak on behalf of God, but I helped people plan for their futures and when they do something wrong, if they violated the law or a Commandment, I help them deal with the consequences."

"Pastor Thomas?"

"Not quite. We both had to go to school for a long time to do what we do and both spend a great deal of time trying to convince others that we are right, you to a congregation, me to jury."

"But, you get paid a great deal more than me."

"That's because I'm selling slop and you're preaching the Gospel. I'm compensated during my lifetime, you're compensated after yours. I'd trade."

"But, what I receive in the hereafter, is available to you as well. I get no more for doing what I do than you receive, if you believe."

"I like your odds better than mine."

"When I was in the seminary, I met some evil and wicked people, people who hoped to shed their sinful ways in the church. Some were successful, others were not. I know a man who preaches in South Carolina, who is mean-spirited and egocentric. I think he stands before his congregation to ingratiate himself, not advance the Lord. Far be it for me to judge, but I suspect he is filled with immorality. And there are priests who have violated the trust of their congregations by sexually abusing children. It's not the collar that gets you into Heaven."

"I'm sure you're right. At 75, dying and in hospice, I guess I'm still a bit naïve."

"Not naïve, respectful of my profession. It's rooted in optimism and faith and I appreciate that. Most of us are good, caring people who chose the profession for the right reasons, but, there are nasty priests and pastors. We all need to be careful, but thank you for your faith."

"My faith wavers while I lay in this bed."

"Mine waivers as well. Faith exists in our hearts and souls. We believe and because we believe, we are faithful. God doesn't confirm our convictions daily with a precisely articulated lesson affirmed with evidence we can see, feel or test. The truth isn't presented with numbers, stones, booming voices from the Heavens or a God who engages in discourse designed to prove his existence and your dependence. Our truth is planted by God in our souls and our hearts and is challenged daily by the evil in the world. When a child dies, we say, *Why?* When a loved one is stricken by cancer, we say, *Why?* When soldiers die on a battlefield, when we are denied our most desired treasures or are ridiculed for our Christian beliefs, we ask *Why?* And when we ask, God does not appear and provide a clear, uncontroverted answer, he asks that we rely on our faith, the spiritual muscle he planted in our hearts and souls when we were baptized. It's hard to deny death, pestilence, pain and hunger, but God gives us the strength to do so. Your faith waivers? Mine does as well."

"If your faith waivers, how are you so sure?"

"I'm not. I believe, I'm not certain. I don't think anyone is. Maintaining belief in spite of all of the reasons to discard it, is a testament to our Christian faith."

"So, I'm not lost because I'm unsure?"

"No. You are found because you are unsure, yet believe."

"Complicated."

"Like the law. The legislature passes a simple law and appellate courts write hundreds of pages trying to make that law clear, and sometimes, they can't. God's word, the Bible, hundreds of pages long, yet scholars and men and women of faith have filled libraries trying to make it clear, and sometimes, they can't. You're right, complicated."

Paul had decided to forgo confession when his confession was to be directed to Mary, but thought that confessing to Pastor James might accomplish the same goal without creating a similar disturbance. "Catholics confess their sins to their priests and are asked to make penance and, as a result, are forgiven for their transgressions. Lutherans don't have confessionals. Do you receive confessions?"

"Our Church believes that your sins are between you and God. You are forgiven when you confess your sins to God and ask for his forgiveness. I'm not a necessary party. Jesus died for your sins. If you believe, if you confess your sins, Jesus' death on the Cross and his resurrection, assures forgiveness and everlasting life."

"That seems a bit simple. No embarrassment, no humility. Too easy."

"God doesn't require that you embarrass yourself to another man, to obtain forgiveness. It's not about your relationship with me or any other man or woman, it's about your relationship with God. I can't forgive you, only God can forgive you and because Jesus died on the Cross, he will forgive you if you believe, confess your sins to him and ask for forgiveness."

"In writing? On my knees? In a church while sitting in a pew?"

"Anywhere, in any manner. So long as it is sincere, the place and manner do not matter."

"You're good."

"What do you mean?"

"I sat in Sunday School for years and in Church for decades and didn't understand. In five minutes, you've taught me most of what I now know about sin, confession, the resurrection and forgiveness. And you made it all clear wearing running shoes and shorts not a robe or clerical collar."

"I take no credit. You've heard what I've said many times before. And I'm sure, it's been said more clearly. The difference isn't me, it's you."

"I haven't changed."

"Yes, you have. You are in bed, dying. The lesson is more important now. Its impact is more immediate. You're willing."

Paul smiled. His smile wasn't mischievous or insincere. She was right. He was willing. He wanted her to leave, so he could have a conversation with God. He had been told what he needed to do and was more than ready to do it. Paul offered Pastor James his disappearing right paw and said, "Thank you. In spite of your humility, or maybe because of it, you have done a yeoman's job. I understand and appreciate it. Thank you."

"You're welcome. I'm glad I could help."

As she turned to leave her church which doubled as Paul's hospice, Paul said, "Tell Mary and the kids to give me a minute. I'm going to have a conversation with God."

"Prayer, Paul, prayer."

"Thanks Pastor."

Before she crossed the threshold, as her feet sounded in the hall, Paul closed his eyes and moved his lips, lowering his guard and confessing his sins. When he heard Mary walk into the room five minutes later, he opened his eyes, refreshed and forgiven. "She's a good person. A heck of a minister."

chapter twenty four

Paul hoped that his theory of the everlasting had merit. After five minutes alone with God, he felt good about the life he lived. He had made mistakes, but he had confessed and atoned for those errors and was guilt free, absolved by one of the two that counted. Recognizing he could not seek forgiveness from the other one that mattered, Mary, he accepted what he had, and felt unburdened from his errors. He was ready.

Paul's trek from Hell to salvation was inspiring, but tiring. When he contemplated an eternity of pain brought on by his indiscretion, he was anxious and when the tension disappeared after a conversation with God, *prayer* as Pastor James called it, and was replaced by peace, his body relaxed and melted into the mattress that supported him. Relieved, relaxed and resurrected, he was tired, very tired.

"Mary, I'm tired. Can you tell the kids I need a nap?"

Before Mary could answer, Paul's eyes closed and his breathing became quiet, shallow and slow. The sleep of an almost dead, yet guilt-free man. Mary tapped his hand, kissed his forehead, wiped the table clean with the wash rag she carried and walked out of the room with a smile on her face.

Paul dreamed. He walked down his long driveway, kicking migrant stones off the tar and into the ditches from which they came. The deported rocks rolled down hills filled with thistle and grasses and nestled in clover that grew where water pooled after rains. Paul raised his collar to protect his neck from November winds which blew in December snows, snows that would soon be cleared by a 38 inch snow blower that was allergic to migrant rocks. Anticipating snow, protecting his snow blower, Paul kicked the driveway clean and listened as the rocks tumbled and died in the soft ditch.

When he reached the road, Seventh Avenue, he turned and walked towards his house a hundred yards away. On the left side of the driveway, 30 yards from and in front of his house, Paul saw an outbuilding he hadn't seen before. He'd lived on Seventh Avenue for 20 years, yet hadn't noticed the building before. It wasn't hidden by vegetation; its visibility not compromised by a hill, a deck or play-set. It was evident, stark, unobstructed, yet previously unseen. *What the hell? Hmm.*

The building was small and dilapidated. The roof was warped and the shingles curled and separated, revealing mold covered, rotting plywood. The windows were broken and the building's siding was moisture laden and soft. Paul walked to the door of the shed and opened it, and as he did, a 50 gallon metal drum attached to a large pump with pipes that pierced the floor of the shed and burrowed through the dirt below, broke free from the pipes and pump and tipped toward Paul, threatening his safety. Paul caught the drum, returned it to its former resting spot and asked himself, *Why haven't I noticed this place before?*

Paul stepped outside and circumnavigated the small shed's outside perimeter, and when he returned to the door, he stepped inside. The interior had grown while Paul had walked around the shanty's exterior. The pump, and metal drum that held water extracted from the ground by the pump, the barrel that tipped and threatened Paul, were gone, and in its place, a fireplace grew from the floor and extended to the now high ceiling. On the far wall, thirty feet from the door where Paul stood, a two basin sink, stove and refrigerator stood beneath a large window that looked into the woods that formed a sleeve on the meandering driveway. Wet, yet inviting and functional furniture, rested in the large open space between Paul and the kitchen, waiting for dry weather, protection from the rain and human contact.

It was a guest cottage. It was neglected and in need of repair, but its potential was evident. Paul turned and surveyed his discovery. *Wow! This is great. How could I have lived here, thirty yards from this building and never have noticed it?*

A gust of wind rattled the cottage and exposed holes in the walls and roof. *Potential. This place has potential and it's mine. I have no talent, but I can read, I can learn. I am retiring. I can commit myself to this building, to restoring it to its original state, when it was warmed by a fireplace and provided shelter to those who entered. I'll buy table saws, power tools, plywood, wood-screws, shingles, paint, cleansers to kill the mold, carpet and lighting. I'll do it. My discovery will become my purpose.*

Paul walked toward the kitchen on the far wall and as he did, he passed books and plans resting on a table with peeling veneer. Although the table had been nearly destroyed by water that entered the cottage through holes in the ceiling, the books and plans were unaffected by nature. They were dry, flat and readable. They were signed by a familiar name, the name of the man from whom Paul had purchased the property, Phil Watson. *I'll call Phil Watson, find out what this property was like when it was built and I'll do everything I can to restore it to its original condition.*

Paul stepped outside the cottage and walked down the driveway, away from the cottage and his home, toward Seventh Avenue, to get a better look at what he had just discovered. He turned, looked towards his new discovery and the house, and was flabbergasted. His house looked so different than it had, before Paul discovered its sibling. The cottage, a garnish to the main course, little sister to the Homecoming Queen, changed the house's appearance, making it bigger, more imposing, elegant. Paul was breathless, impressed. *Wow! When I'm done, maybe I'll live in the cottage and rent the house to royalty. Sweet.*

As Paul began to make a mental list, *a table saw, plywood, Sawzall, shingles,* a pan in the kitchen fell loudly to the floor and startled, Paul opened his eyes. He looked out the open window, searching for his cottage, his purpose, but it wasn't there. It had disappeared as quickly as it had appeared. He looked around the room and saw a box of rubber gloves, an inter-venous bag on a tall pole, bedding folded and stored on the top of a bed stand, a metal tray clogged with bottles of pills and his bed, a hospital bed with side-rails to keep the sick in bed. The cottage was gone;

the future of which he dreamed was dead. No cottage, no shed, no wherewithal to leave his bed and complete a project and paint a dream. Alone and unable, Paul cried.

Paul didn't shed tears because he would soon succumb to cancer; the tears were shed because his condition was ever-present and unrelenting. He wasn't in pain, wasn't afraid of dying or what he would face when the curtain descended. He was diminished and hurt, because if a shed needed his attention, he was unable to provide it, now or ever.

Cancer would take his life. He'd be dead. Gone. *Okay. Understood.* But, sheds would need repair and he couldn't repair them. His grandchildren would grow older, fall in love and marry and he wouldn't be able to judge their choices, counsel them or attend the weddings. Trump could be on the ballot, but he couldn't cast a vote in favor of his opponent, no matter who that opponent was. Rocks would need to be cleared from his driveway when the cold weather reappeared, and it always did, but he wouldn't be able to survey the tar or kick rocks to the ditch. In the future, a doctor would tell Mary that her long life would soon end, but he wouldn't be there to comfort her, to tell her it was okay, that it was inevitable, but not painful or demon-filled.

Paul didn't cry because he was in pain or would soon die, he shed tears because he understood others would live and that he would not be there to share their lives with them. The shed would remain dilapidated, Mary would die without his comfort, his grandchildren would grow old without him around, rocks would either damage machinery or be kicked to the curb by boots worn by someone other than Paul and Trump could be elected without his dissenting ballot.

343

When Paul wiped tears from his eyes, he looked to the doorway and saw Aly standing at the threshold with a pot in hand. "Sorry Dad. It fell. It was loud. Sorry."

Paul smiled. "I thought we were under attack."

"Were you crying?"

"A little."

"Why?"

"I won't be able to restore the cottage."

"What cottage?"

"Never mind." Paul wiped a tear from a cheek, cleared his throat and answered the question Aly asked. "It'll be over soon. I won't be able to go to Joe's wedding. I can't hold your Mom's hand when she is in this bed. Can't say *No* to Trump. Life will go on, and I won't be here to help when I'm needed. I won't be able to share in your joy or make you laugh. I want to be there, to count, to contribute." Realizing that death's pain was compounded by the continuing lives of survivors, tears fell from Paul's eyes to his pillow. "You'll be here, I won't."

Aly walked to her Dad, put the noisy pot on the end of the bed where the side-rails assured that it would not fall and disturb the quiet, and took Paul's hands in hers. She whispered. "You'll be here. We'll keep going, because of you. When we laugh, we'll remember your laugh and when the laughter stops, we'll tell stories about you, about us, and we'll laugh again. When Joe finds the right woman, the woman he chooses to marry, he'll remember the advice you gave him when you fished on Green Lake and he asked you why you married Grandma. If Trump is elected, he will be challenged, questioned and held accountable by those who have been influenced by your words. Clients you have helped will live their lives happier and more complete, because of what you've done. You have impacted this world in many different ways, through your practice, your service, your friends and your family. You'll be dead, but you'll still be here."

"But, who'll restore the cottage?"

"What cottage?"

"Never mind."

Aly sat on the chair, next to her Father's bed. Without a book, magazine, television, radio, phone or iPad, her mind was clear, unobstructed. Typically, allergic to stillness, silence, Aly sat quietly, listening to her Dad breathe. She was there, always would be. When his eyes closed and a smile graced his peaceful face, she knew she had done what needed to be done. *The truth set us free.*

While Paul slept, Joe introduced him to his fiancé and Paul approved. While Paul slept, he cleaned the shed, patched holes, re-roofed, reinforced the foundation and painted the walls white. While Paul slept, he stood on the Capital steps and explained to thousands, maybe millions, why it would be a mistake to elect an egocentric, immature, dishonest, sociopath, president. While he slept, Paul watched over what he'd leave behind and felt his presence even after he was gone. As Paul slept, he smiled.

chapter twenty five

*P*aul was never a good fisherman. He was an adequate angler, a man who could bait a hook, toss it in the water, and if a fish found it, could turn the crank and reel it in. But if the fish weren't biting, had moved from his favorite hole or were nibbling, not biting, flirting, not screwing, his live-well remained empty.

Paul was never much of a hunter. His dad took him into the woods when he was an old child or very young adult, and educated him on the skills necessary to kill the potentially delicious ruffed-tailed grouse, but when he nearly stepped on one in the woods, rather than flush it and shoot while it flew away, Paul shot it where it stood and transformed a potentially good meal into feathers, obliterated meat and shotgun shell pellets. He hunted deer from when he was 12 until 40, and although he trudged through cold and snow in November, and sat quietly in a tree while his teeth chattered and his feet froze, he had only killed one deer, a fawn he shot while aiming at its mother.

Paul liked to watch hockey, but had never played. He turned on the television on Saturdays and watched Gopher football, was happy when they won and sad when they lost, but he didn't know the difference between a tackle and a guard, a safety and a touchback, a tailback and a half-back or a four-three and a three-four, and had never played the game.

Paul fought in a war, but wasn't a warrior. When a Vietcong sniper's rifle sounded with a *pop, pop, pop,* Paul was the first of his squad to find cover, when they came upon a disfigured NVA, killed by a booby-trap on a trail through the jungle, Paul stood silently and watched as others from his squadron pulled it clear so they could pass. And although he was offended, angry and encouraged by testosterone to stand and fight when someone spoke badly of him, his family or friends, he never clenched his fists, squared off or threw a punch.

He spent time in a boat with a pole in his hands. He spent time in the woods with a firearm in his hands. He was a casual observer of athletes, not an athlete. He contributed to the war effort, without getting bloody or bruised.

His life was lived on the sidelines. He was a high school letter winner, an angler and hunter and a Vietnam veteran; however, he'd not caught the winning touchdown, bagged a trophy walleye or 16-point buck or worn a Purple-heart on his chest.

Awake, laying in a bed with side-rails, lifted and locked in place, to keep the sick in bed, likely hours or days from death he asked, *Did I do enough? Did I show enough courage? Was I afraid and because of my fears, reluctant to do what needed to be done?*

When Tom Dahlheimer goaded me and punched me, should I have punched him back? I didn't. Was I a chicken, afraid to do what should have been done? When the sniper's bullets sounded and I hid, should I have scanned the tree-tops in search of the enemy and shot him dead? I didn't. Was I afraid and exposing my friends to danger by not rising above my fears? When my dad asked me to try out for the football team or get back on the ice after falling and hitting my head, when I said No, was I simply small and frightened, and if I had done as suggested, would I have learned that effort, competition, teamwork and bruises branded on a field of play, transform a boy into a man, and a chicken into a brave soul? Did I do enough? Was I brave enough?

Lonnie Hatton was 82 pounds in seventh grade, the smallest boy in Paul's gym class. His hair was red, his eyes blue, his feet large and his enthusiasm, unmistakable. When the gym teacher said, *Today, we're going to play volleyball,* Lonnie jumped high, smiled ear-to-ear, pumped his small fists into the air, squealed and shouted, *Great!* When the gym teacher said, *Today, we're going to wrestle,* Lonnie jumped high, smiled ear-to-ear, pumped his small fists into the air, squealed and shouted, *Great!* When the gym teacher said, *Today, we're going to square dance,* Lonnie jumped high, smiled ear-to-ear, pumped his small fists into the air, squealed and shouted, *Great!*

Lonnie was fearless. When asked to pick an opponent to wrestle, he chose the biggest, strongest boy in class, and when asked to pick a position to play on the volleyball court, he chose the front-line, middle spot where spikers typically rose above the net and drove the ball down for a point, even though Lonnie could not lift himself to touch the net, let alone rise above it. He enthusiastically rode the bench on the football squad and the hockey team and ran track in the fall, where he almost always finished each race last, with a smile on his face. When bigger boys, malcontents, threatened or embarrassed him, he lifted his popcorn fists and fought, until he was bloody and unable to continue or a teacher or cop said, *That's enough.*

Lonnie didn't wait to be drafted. He enlisted before graduating from high school and was in basic training before hangovers from after-graduation parties lifted themselves from bigger, stronger, smarter classmates. He was in Vietnam before his nineteenth birthday and brought home in a box two-months after he arrived.

In bed, dying, Paul asked again, *Was I brave enough? Lonnie Hatton was. He was unafraid. He accepted challenges without being concerned about the consequences. He played hard, he fought hard and he died young, before he could fall in love, before he could sire children, before he could relax on a beach, in a lounge chair, with a beer in his hands. Dead, but not forgotten. I remember. He only lived 19 years, but was his life more consequential than mine? He was unbridled, not shackled by fear. He died a man. Nineteen, yet old and wise and dead.*

Should I have asked to sing a solo? Should I have volunteered to debate the Principal on the dress code? Should I have practiced the trumpet and played challenging melodies rather than drift to the tuba to play pedantic oomp pahs? When the captain asked for a volunteer, should I have raised my hand? Did I try enough cases? Did I fight when it was easier to walk away? Did I accept life's challenges, in spite of the consequences? Did I do everything I could have done? Was I Chicken Little or Lonnie Hatton?

It's too late to change now. I'll never know the thrill Lonnie knew when the gym teacher said, Today, it's volleyball. I'll never know if he was afraid when he lifted his fists, knowing his face would soon be bloodied and bruised. I'll never know if he found peace in death, knowing he had lived his life, free from compunctions and full of risks and rewards. Lonnie wore a badge of fearlessness on his face after being pummeled, but he died a teenager, childless, in a place far from home. Lonnie made choices consistent with who he was and died because of those choices. I cautiously ambulated from childhood, to adulthood to a hospice bed. I was fearful, but my fears protected me and delivered me three children, a devoted wife and 75 years of making a small difference. Well done, Lonnie. You have my undying respect and admiration. Well done. But, I'm not you and never was, and after careful consideration, I'm okay with that. Hold the door, my friend, I'm coming.

"Welcome back. Sleep well?"

Mary stood at the end of the bed with side-rails, wearing shorts, sandals, a tank-top and Noxzema on her nose. Paul smiled, knowing Lonnie never knew Mary or how a man could feel about the love of his life. Like almost always, Mary had ended the inquiry with an articulate, wordless answer. Fearlessness had killed Lonnie and fear had given Paul the time to love Mary.

"You know they have sunscreen to do what Noxzema did when we were young."

"I know. Old habits die hard."

As Mary wiped the white oil from her nose, Paul watched and smiled.

chapter twenty six

*H*ad he lived, Paul's brother would have been 69. He died without taking a breath and was buried without a name. After his death, his still-birth, his near birth, his parents never spoke of him and the room remodeled to be his bedroom, filled with boxes, unused furniture, old newspapers, was forever dark, imprisoned in blackness by permanently drawn curtains. He disappeared before he appeared. One day he was anticipated and the next, nearly forgotten.

They forgot; I could not. It wasn't so easy for a six year old boy.

Two days before Thanksgiving in 1946, Paul's mother walked into Paul's bedroom and said, "The rabbit died." Paul had no idea what a dead rabbit meant, but by what he saw, it must have been a good thing. His mother's cheeks were red, without blush, her eyes bright and clear and her smile broad. "Do you know what that means, Paul? When I say the rabbit died, do you know what that means?"

Paul didn't and said so.

"It means, I'm going to have baby and you're going to have a baby brother or sister."

It didn't register immediately. Things were good for Paul and change not anticipated was unwelcome. It had always been just Paul and his parents. Just Paul. He rode in the car between his mom and dad and the backseat was empty. If he woke in the night frightened by a nightmare, his cries woke no one but his mom and dad and after being comforted by the only other two in the home, he slept in his parents' bed while the rest of the house was quiet and unoccupied. When they sat in a pew at church, there were three Thomases, not four and when doctors, teachers, strangers in need of small talk topics and new friends asked Paul to describe his family, he said, *Mom, Dad and me, that's it. Just us.*

"Are you excited, Paul? A brother or sister. Won't it be fun?"

The backseat? No room on their bed for me? Share? Someone else? Not just me? Paul said nothing.

Because her question didn't elicit the answer she had hoped for, she changed it into a statement. "Paul, it'll be fun."

"What's for lunch?"

"Whatever you want, sweetie."

Resistance diminished as Paul's mother's stomach grew. Ahead of their time, Sixties parents in 1946, Paul's parents understood that the new arrival would increase the size of their family, and mathematically diminish Paul's role in the family and further understood, that although Paul couldn't explain the mathematic consequences, he knew he'd be relatively less when the family became more. To counteract Paul's concerns, to help him better understand that sometimes more meant more, his Mom and Dad shared their journey with him, involving him in it, to the extent they could. He was told about doctor visits and asked if he had questions for the doctor. He was told that they would name the child as a family and was asked for name recommendations for both a brother and a sister. When the storage room was emptied and cleaned and converted into a child's bedroom, Paul helped and picked out the wallpaper that would greet his newborn sibling each morning after sleep. He put his ear to his mother's protruded belly and felt his brother, his sister, move, attempting to escape confinement and join Paul for play.

It worked. Paul was excited. He accepted his diminished role in the household, happily accepting a more important role as a brother, mentor and protector. As his mother's stomach blossomed, his excitement grew. He spent sleepless nights in bed, wearing a smile, daydreaming in the dark about his brother wearing a baseball glove too big for his small hands or his sister pouring imaginary tea into imaginary tea cups. He rose from bed after sleepless nights, tired yet happy. Anticipation. He was excited.

On June 4, 1947, Paul lifted himself from his bed and walked down the stairs to the kitchen. His mom was not at the stove, his grandmother, Paul's father's mother was. She turned to face Paul, smiled broadly, grandmotherly, and said, "Your mom and dad are at the hospital. You're going to have a brother or sister later today."

At 4:00 p.m., Paul's grandmother answered the telephone with a smile of anticipation, and after few words, returned the phone to its cradle, wearing a grimace and a tear in her eye. Recognizing that joy had been drawn from the room by a telephone call, Paul asked, "What Grandma? What?"

After being told he would need to wait until his dad came home, Paul went to his bedroom, where a pall converted daydreams to daymares. The radio in the living room was silent, the phone didn't ring, Grandma didn't talk, neither did Paul.

When Paul's dad came home, rather than greet him at the door as he always did, Paul apprehensively waited for him in his bedroom. After closing the door to the baby's bedroom, his dad, visibly broken, wearing a rumpled white shirt, loosely knotted black tie and stained black pants and scuffed shoes, walked down the hall, stood in Paul's bedroom doorway, gripped the door frame with his left hand and said, "Your brother died. He won't be coming home. Sorry."

The joy was gone, the door to the baby's room remained closed and silence plagued the home. Paul's mother returned from the hospital three days after his brother died without living, and his father returned to his restaurant two days thereafter. For nearly two weeks after his mom returned home, she said almost nothing. The radio remained off, and telephone calls were frequent, but telephone conversations, short. His mother answered the calls and ended each with a somber whisper, *Thank you.*

When school began in September, the drape of death was raised by time and shards of light and hope began creeping into Paul's home. His mom turned on the radio, hummed with Sinatra and asked Paul if he liked first grade. When he told her did, for the first time in months, Paul saw her smile.

It snowed two days before Christmas and the Thomas family, Paul, Mom and Dad, shoveled the walk, built a snowman and warmed chilly bones, standing near the kitchen radiator, drinking hot milk. They laughed, they talked about Santa Claus, they teased each other, smiled, hugged and sang a Christmas song. That night, Paul woke when an imaginary dragon took hold of his sleeping left foot. He cried out and his mom rescued him and brought him to their bed, where he slept soundly, between Mom and Dad, not disturbing anyone but his mom and dad. Two days later, Paul rode to church in the front seat of a panel van branded with a hand painted sign advertising *Hi-Way 10 Café*. The van's back seat was empty and when they arrived at church, the three, not four, three members of the Thomas household sat in a pew and listened to the Pastor celebrate the birth of Christ. As the small family walked from the nave to the narthex, Pastor Rust, shook Paul's Dad's hand, smiled and said, *The Thomas family. Have a blessed Christmas.* He smiled at Paul, took the hand of Paul's mother in his and smiled. The smile was not joyful, not celebratory, but obviously, compassionate and sympathetic. He nodded as the family of three, Paul, his mom and his dad, walked from the church into the Minnesota cold.

Paul didn't know what happened at the hospital, he never asked, and his parents never offered. Paul didn't know if the grief that swallowed his family during the summer of 1947, shattered his parents' dreams of a larger family, he never asked and they never offered. They moved on and by 1948, it seemed to Paul like his parents had forgotten what had inspired hope and joy and dealt grief and remorse.

Paul never forgot. The memory never died. At six, he was unable to move on without lingering questions or haunting visions. He couldn't forget. He remembered what was supposed to be and didn't understand why it wasn't. As a primary school boy, Paul dreamed of his brother. The dream was persistent, consistent. Paul's imagination, fostered by seven months of anticipation, seven months of listening to his brother attempt to break free from gestation and into life, seven months of preparation for what wouldn't be, was vivid and created something nearly palpable. He dreamed and when his dream was coupled with intense desire, he saw. He saw his brother.

He was Paul's friend, his protectorate, confidant and a lover of dogs, baseball, Elvis and cool mornings in August. He was studious and quiet, mischievous and supportive, honest and smart. He rarely found trouble, and if he did, Paul shouldered the consequences without involving him. He was always there, always willing, almost always smiling. When he was conceived by Paul, when he first appeared, he was dead only five days, but in Paul's mind, he weighed 40 pounds, sat upright and straight on the end of Paul's twin bed, wore a white shirt, with black pants and a black tie, and while he waited for Paul to speak, gently kicked his feet as they hung from the bed, attached to his short legs, two feet from the floor. He waited. And waited.

Although he rarely spoke his name out loud, Paul named him, doing something his grief filled parents were unable to do after the doctor said, *I'm sorry*. He named him Bill.

Bill understood Paul as no one else did. He was always there, always willing to console, always supportive. He was, as Paul wanted him to be.

Bill helped Paul find perspective and combat ever present doom that often visited boys not yet old enough to shave. When life said *Boo*, Paul jumped and often needed calming. Childhood. Challenges. Coping. Paul needed help and Bill provided that help. When Paul contracted measles, and was bed-ridden for 10 days in 1948, Bill sat quietly on the end of the bed and offered hope when Paul wondered if he would succumb to the germs or battle, win and return to the field of play. *What are you worried about? I'm dead, you're just fighting a very beatable childhood disease. Toughen up.* When Paul was unable to sleep, fretting about singing alone in front of his fifth-grade class, Bill said, *It won't kill you. Look at me, consider the options and lighten up.* When Angela Thompson told Paul she had no intention of going to the sixth grade dance with him, that she was likely in love with a seventh grader, when Paul responded with tears, Bill, sitting on the end of the bed, still wearing black pants, a white shirt and tie, spotted by dog fur, said, *At least some day you'll dance, not me. I'm dead, or at least unalive. Relax a bit.*

They communicated as brothers often do, secretly, without spoken, audible words, but rather with magic, silence and telepathy. In the dark, when only furnaces, the refrigerator and toilets with faulty washers ran, or in the light, when boys ran after girls and dogs after squirrels, Bill kept watch over his brother. When Paul was troubled, Bill was there, when Paul wanted to celebrate an accomplishment, Bill was there, when Paul needed reassurance, direction or hope, he was there. Paul laid on his bed and silently asked his brother for help and so long as he was needed, Bill was there and always provided the answer Paul sought.

And then, he was gone. There was no warning, no premonition, no writing on the wall. He was just gone.

Paul failed an eighth grade science test, was told that he could do better and if he didn't, he would repeat eighth grade. Despondent and scared, wary that high school graduation could be delayed and that he might graduate with the seventh grade twerps he passed in the halls of his junior high, little kids whose voices were high and experience low, Paul labored into his bedroom, sat on the bed and looked for Bill, for encouragement and hope, but he wasn't there. Paul spoke his name, *Bill*, but he wasn't there, didn't respond.

Paul opened his *Natural Science* book, studied it, asked scientific questions, found scientific answers, took notes about what he read, highlighted important information in the text and reviewed the notes and highlights before the next test. After the test, when Mr. Steadman returned graded tests to Paul's classmates, he withheld Paul's and said, "Mr. Thomas, I'd like to meet with you after class to talk about your test."

When the bell rang, signaling the end of Science class, Paul slouched in his chair and waited to be told that little kids with high voices and little experience would soon be his classmates, but instead, Mr. Steadman said, "Well done young man. From an F to a perfect test. Keep up the good work."

At the end of the school day, with the corners of his mouth near his ears, Paul rushed from class and through the crowded doorway, bumping into seventh graders and passing them wearing a superior scowl and ran home to share his test with his mom and dad. After he did, he went to his bedroom to tell Bill, but when he walked through the door, Bill was not there. And that's when Paul understood, that likely he was gone forever.

Bill was never real. Paul knew that. Bill had a name, a place to live, answers when questions were asked, a white shirt, black tie and pants, but Paul knew he wasn't real. He didn't wake Paul's mom and dad with his whispers late at night or leave an impression on the bed where he sat. He didn't leave the bed to use the bathroom, never grew and never changed his clothes. Paul knew he wasn't real, but he was something Paul needed, and when he didn't need him anymore, he was gone. Curiosity killed the cat, Oswald killed Kennedy and Paul's maturity killed Bill. Older, more able, capable of fending for himself and beating back challenges with hard work, maturity and experience, Paul no longer needed to rely on Bill, and for the second time in his nonexistent life, Bill died.

As he laid in a bed, protected from the floor by side-rails designed to keep the sick in bed, Paul wondered if Bill would be a guide when he died and the world in which he had lived for more than 75 years vanished and he needed someone to show him the way. *Will he wear a black tie, a white shirt and black pants? Will he be as I pictured him, will he be what he would have been had he been born and lived 69 years, or will he be an oxygen starved infant deprived of life?*

"Mary, did I tell you I named my brother?"

"No. We were married for thirty years before you told me you had a brother. You are talking about the brother who was still-born?"

"Yup. He was the only one. I named him Bill."

"Why?"

"No one else did. Seeing all that he was missing, not living and all, I thought it was the least I could do. He'd never have a wife or kids, never have a car or house, I thought at least he should have a name."

"Why Bill?"

"I don't remember. I was six. It was a long time ago. Maybe I watched a Wild Bill Hickok the day before I named him. Maybe I'd heard Buffalo Bill with Howdy Doodey the day before I named him. I don't know."

"It was Buffalo Bob. Not Bill."

"Well then it wouldn't have been because I watched Buffalo *Bill* with Howdy Doodey. Maybe I heard about Buffalo Bill Cody on the radio. I don't know. It was 69 years ago. I named him Bill and can't remember why."

Mary stood, lightly gripped the bed side-rail that was a barrier between Paul and the chair in which she had sat, and asked, "Why bring up your still-born brother?"

Paul smiled. The grin across his face remained as he answered Mary's question. "I won't golf again. You're still a beautiful woman, but I'll never sleep with you again. I won't hit tennis balls with Lauren again and I doubt I'll ever leave this room to watch the sun rise or set, or feel a gentle warm breeze on my face. I don't have much to look forward to."

"What does that have to do with your brother."

"I waited seven months to see him and have waited another 69 years. My wait may be over. Maybe I'll see him soon. It's something I'm looking forward to." His smile remained.

Paul closed his eyes and when desire fortified imagination, as he softly breathed in and out and his chest rose and fell, he saw him. Bill. He sat on the end of Paul's bed, wearing black pants, a white shirt and black tie. He smiled and with his smile, comforted the man once six, now 75, the man once young, now old. And at peace and not alone, Paul slept.

chapter twenty seven

Paul dreamed. It was election Tuesday. 2016. Paul followed his brother Bill to the polling place in the living room of Paul's home.

The Election Judge wore a smile, a red button that read *I Voted,* and spoke in an Eastern European accent. She handed Paul a ballot, pointed to a voting booth across the living room, near the kitchen table where Paul and his children shared meals of meatloaf, lasagna, hot-dish and pizza, and said, *Go. Vote. Do as you are to do. Vote.*

As Paul pulled the booth's curtain open, he heard Bill argue with the Czechoslovakian Election Judge, an argument that ended when the Eastern European barked, *You can't vote, you didn't even live. Out. You're not velcome here. Immigrants. There ought to be a wall to keep the still-born out. Immigrants. Rapists, killers, still-born immigrants. Huh! Out!*

Paul, the six-year old boy, the 75 year old cancer patient with wrinkled skin and thinning hair, wanted to flee the polling place and wrap his brother in his arms and salve the wounds inflicted in the womb and in the living room occupied by an Eastern European election judge who was incapable of compassion and unwilling to sympathize with the still-born, but before he could pursue justice, the Czechoslovakian disappeared and Bill laid in a stroller, wearing diapers, sucking a pacifier. Like Bill's life, the battle ended before it began.

Confused, but recognizing a confrontation had been avoided and he was free to do what people do when they vote, choose between candidates to determine those best suited to govern, Paul walked into the booth and looked at his ballot. There were 122 races on the eighteen-page ballot, for offices from Public Service Officer/Dog Catcher to President of the United States. *Choices. So many choices.* And then Paul noticed the candidates for every office, for dog catcher to president and everything in between, the ones noted as Democrat, Republican, Communist, Independent, Socialist and Libertarian, were all the same man. *One. No other choice.*

Enraged, Paul crumpled his ballot into a ball, a large ball, a ball the size of a twelve-pound medicine ball and stormed to the table occupied by election judges, six overweight, orange-faced men, with bronzed cotton candy hair and confused blue eyes and bellered, *What's this?*, but before they could answer, like the Czechoslovakian, they disappeared.

Alone, Paul returned to his bedroom and saw Bill sitting on the end of his bed in a crease he earlier created, wearing a white shirt, black pants and a black tie. A hairless old man with sharp bones shook beneath the white cotton sheets of the bed where

Bill sat. Paul ran to the bed, pulled the sheets from the elderly man and discovered he was bronzed, with no hair. The old boney man smiled, revealing puffy gums and brown teeth and said, *Did you vote for me?*

Paul took a deep, sharp breath and opened his eyes. No boney old man, no Bill, no polling booth, no election judges. *Just Mary.* Groggy, confused, desperate, agitated, *still asleep,* Paul pleaded with Mary. "Evil. You've gotta stop evil. It's a nightmare. We need to stop it before it's too late, before it becomes the only option."

Mary grinned. "Why would it become the only option?"

"In my nightmares, it can't tolerate competition. Give it a foothold and it'll do everything it can to eliminate the competition, and once it's gone, it's the only option. Promise me, after I'm gone, you'll do what you can to protect our children and their future from that vile creature. Promise me. Please."

Mary grinned and sneered. "Oh. It's not so bad. Lighten up." Mary cleared her throat and scratched the top of her head with an arm that grew from her back, in between sharp shoulder blades and above her tail.

Paul took a deeper, sharper breath and opened his eyes, *really* opened his eyes and ended the nightmare within a nightmare. No boney old man, no Bill, no polling booth, no election judges no third arm in Marys back, just Mary as she was on the day they married, except a little bit older.

Paul wanted to be sure. *Am I awake?* "Turn around please." When Mary did and Paul saw her tail was gone and her third arm only a nightmarish memory, he said, "Thanks. A nightmare in the middle of the day. The drugs deaden the pain, but sharpen the imagination."

"What was it about? The nightmare?"

"Nothing important. Power and the need to maintain it. Unimportant. Let's just keep it that way."

While Mary plumped up pillows, changed towels, freshened water and wiped dried tears from Paul's salty cheeks, Paul contemplated his legacy. His nightmare within a nightmare, his dark dream in the middle of the day, his foray into the future with evil at the helm, startled him and he asked himself, *What have I done to protect the future from evil? Enough?*

Paul had been urged to run for the School Board when his children were in elementary school, but didn't. When his State Legislative Representative was arrested on stalking charges and surprisingly entered the next election unopposed, Paul considered mounting a campaign to unseat him, but didn't. When Paul Wellstone died and one of Minnesota's Senate seats were unoccupied, he thought of standing before the voters and professing his love for progressive politics and attempting to replace a man he admired, but didn't. And *now*, when Trump was dominating the headlines, when polling numbers showed him to be the front runner, when Paul found it unacceptable to elect an unsuccessful business man, a man the left labeled as a madman, the leader of the free world, there was little if anything he could do. He was dying. He couldn't fight.

"I should have done more."

Mary put water in a vase that held a bouquet of flowers sent by the Minnesota State Bar Association with a card that read, *Thanks for everything*, set the watering can on the table and asked, "More about what?"

"The world. I held the microphone, but didn't speak. Things needed to be said and I said nothing."

"What do you wish you'd have said?"

"That things could be better. That accepting what was proposed wasn't good enough. That hard work, an open mind and a commitment to excellence would help deliver what we are looking for."

"And what do you think we are looking for?"

"Good health. Clean air and water. Jobs that pay a living wage. Affordable housing. Dignity. Respect. Equal opportunity."

"Those are things most people want, but a quiet lawyer working hard to raise his family and protect his clients doesn't often deliver health care, clean water, affordable housing or equal opportunity."

Paul stared out the window of his cage constructed by cancer, looking beyond Anoka and to the east. He had lived his life where he was born. His hometown was comfortable, his home large, solid, and like his hometown, comfortable. His life had been easy. He hadn't accepted challenges that called from beyond his home, beyond his hometown. He met people on his way to work who knew his name, people who had gone to school with his

children, had eaten meals at his father's restaurant. His clients were locals, classmates, former teammates, teachers, barbers and bankers. The judges before whom he had appeared, knew his name before he spoke and he exchanged Christmas cards with the bailiffs, court clerks, prosecutors and many of the defendants. It had all been too parochial, too safe, way too easy.

"You're right. I was a quiet lawyer, working in a quiet, comfortable town, the town in which I was raised. I fixed little things, but didn't tackle the arduous, the important, the uncomfortable. I had talent and let my talent go to waste."

"You didn't waste your talents. If you believe that, you're crazy."

"No, I think I'm right. I represented the guy that stole food to feed his family, but I didn't propose legislation that would have helped him feed his family legally. I represented dispossessed tenants, but didn't lobby my legislator to introduce legislation designed to make rents more affordable. When a client was sentenced to prison for possessing marijuana, I convinced the appellate court to reduce his sentence, but didn't take to the political stage to urge changes to the criminal code that would legalize a relatively benign drug and protect relatively good people from onerous prosecutions. No, I'm right, I didn't do what I could have done. Too easy. Too damn comfortable."

Mary shook her head and placed calloused hands on her hips. "It's too easy to do what you're doing, to say what you're saying now. When you're near the end, it's too easy to reflect, regret and repudiate. You didn't change the direction of Earth's rotation, didn't warm January or prevent the spread of polio in the fifties, but who did? No one. No one did; no one could. Everyone has talents and should do what he can do to use those talents and make the world a better place. I can't sing opera and shouldn't try. I can't square the corners on a wooden box and shouldn't try to construct a home. I never ran a marathon, because my weak ankles and flat feet wouldn't have carried me. But, I made homeless people feel comfortable on cold January nights when all they wanted was warmth, a mattress and friendly smile. I did what I was meant to do, what I could do given my skills and wants. And regardless of what you say now, you did as I did, worked with your talents to make the world a better place."

Paul pointed a shaky index finger at a button, pushed it and the head of the bed rose. When the head of the bed reached 45 degrees, Paul leaned over the side-rail locked in place between Mary and him, and looked at Mary's feet. His eyes left Mary's feet and returned to her blue eyes. He smiled and asked, "When did your ankles weaken and your arches fall?"

Mary laughed and capitalized on Paul's levity. "Flat feet for me, an unwillingness to pander for you."

Although Paul knew what Mary meant, because he wanted to hear it, he asked anyway. "What do you mean, I was unwilling to pander?"

"You know what I mean." He did, she knew he knew, but understood he wanted to hear it, so she said it anyway. "Politicians change the law. Lobbyist influence politicians. Politicians spend their days raising money, begging for support or sitting in committee meetings, bored out of their minds. Lobbyists are whores who buy legislators' favor, to promote what's good or bad, right talents and should do what he can do to use those talents and make the world a better place. I can't sing opera and shouldn't try. I can't square of their minds. Lobbyists are whores who buy legislators' favor, to promote what's good or bad, right or wrong. You didn't want to beg for money. You didn't want to sit in boring meetings all day long and surely, you didn't want to kiss a representative's butt so that he would support whatever cause you're paid to support. So, tell me that you didn't do enough, that you should have been a senator or lobbyist and I'll tell you, you're full of it. You could no more lobby or legislate than I could build a home, run a marathon or sing an opera. We all have regrets; we all think we could've done more, could've been better, but, you did a wonderful job given your God given skills and desires. It was a job well done."

Mary was on a roll and Paul wanted the roll to continue. He wanted to hear that it wasn't a mistake, that his life was worthwhile, that the choices he made were not all wrong. Close to the end, validation was important. Too important. "I could have skipped the boring committee meetings and served only one term, not needing re-election money."

"One term legislators get nothing done. An effective Congressman has seniority and has been around the legislature long enough to know how it works. To make it work, you've got to know how it works, and that takes time. To have significant impact as an elected official, you need to raise money and attend boring meetings. If you don't do both, because you're not playing by the rules, you waste your time and accomplish nothing. You wouldn't have had the gall to call your mother for a donation, let alone hundreds of strangers. When the Chair pounded his gavel, and began to cite Robert's Rules of Order, you'd have been tempted to resign on the spot. It's just not you.

"You did what you were supposed to do. Ask the impoverished tenant allowed to stay in her apartment because of your advocacy. Ask the pot smoker who avoided prison time because of your tenacity. Ask the man who stole to feed his family if he thought you were doing the right thing when you convinced a jury to ignore the evidence and make its decision based on sympathy for a man who was only trying to keep his family alive. Ask them all. And then ask prosecutors why they refuse to advocate for prison when someone is caught with pot. They'll tell you it's because you convinced the Court of Appeals prison for pot was inappropriate. And ask those same prosecutors why they now recommended no-jail, when an impoverished defendant broke the law to save his family. They'll tell you it's because you convinced a jury to nullify the evidence when it faced the option of jail or accommodations for a man trying to keep his family alive. You did what you were supposed to do and had significant impact when doing it. Don't regret what you didn't do, celebrate what you did. You did a lot."

Almost convinced, Paul asked for an exclamation point, a fitting end to a fitting life. "A priest who forgave sin. A doctor who saved lives. A therapist who exorcized dysfunction. They all did more than me. They were important; I tried, but did little." He waited, grim faced with a smile beneath the surface, a smile waiting to be revealed by the words Paul knew Mary would speak.

"Priests are consumed by religiosity and can't marry or have children. Doctors spend their days with infected and dying patients, after devoting a decade of their lives to college and medical school. Therapists plant seeds and patiently wait for results, results that oftentimes don't appear. You wanted to marry and have children, you were unwilling to spend a decade in a lab coat learning about deviated septums and obstructed bowels and don't have the patience to plant therapeutic seeds and wait months or years for harvest. You were born to advocate, to convince and give legal counsel. You're not a priest, doctor or therapist and couldn't have been. It's not you, never was. So, cry in your beer, regret your past, beg for another chance, but keep in mind, if you were given another chance, you'd never do more than what you did. It was a job well done."

Satisfied, convinced, coddled, Paul accepted the praise and resisted the temptation to ask for more. The smile, previously masked by an illegitimate grim face, revealed itself and Paul accepted the praise. "Thanks. I needed that. Laying here, unable to do much, except accept my fate, death, a fate no one wants to accept, I question things I wouldn't otherwise question. The unknown plants fear and fear plants regret. Living without a future is depressing and that depression leads me to question my past. But, I think you're right. I would have been a promiscuous priest, an incompetent doctor and impatient therapist. I would have failed at all of them. I was a good lawyer. It probably worked the way it should have."

"It did. And you should be proud of what you accomplished as a lawyer, but beyond that, what you accomplished as a father, husband and friend. You lived a good life and should be very proud."

"Understood, and I know I've done this before, questioned my worth, but so close to the end, it's time to tally. I can't avoid it. I'm glad you have the cash box, the ability to review the receipts and evaluate my life. You're right, but if I was left to conduct my own evaluation, at this point, standing on the edge, almost touching the other side, I'd not be objective or complimentary. I'm glad you're here to help. Thanks."

Mary took a boney paw in her hands, pressed softly, smiled at her dying husband of 40 years and ended the conversation. "I'm glad to be here, glad I can help. It's been a good ride and I am thankful I was able to enjoy it with you. You are a good man, Paul Thomas, and don't you dare tell yourself otherwise."

Paul suppressed a cough with a swallow, cleared his throat, swallowed what he dislodged, smiled and closed his tired eyes. Satisfied with the life lived, he slept, peacefully, quietly.

$\mathcal{P}$aul drifted from asleep to awake to asleep to awake, over and over. Conscious, unconscious, awake, asleep. *Huh? Oh.* When he slept, he dreamed, in vivid color, interacting with colorful, animated, ancient characters, and when he was awake, he engaged in short confused conversations with Mary, Alyson, Lauren and Randy, conversations that ended abruptly, prematurely, when Paul was drawn to sleep by cancer, medicine and his colorful, fictional characters.

"Dad, are you there?"

"Yup. Sorry. Where were we?"

"You were telling me about your imaginary brother."

"Oh. Bill. White shirt, black pants and a tie. He was still-born…….."

"Dad. Dad. Dad?"

"Good to meet you ma'am. I'm honored and a bit in awe. I've heard and read so much about you. St. Peter in a dress? The Gatekeeper? Six-hundred-fifteen years old and enough wisdom accumulated to answer everyone's everything?"

She didn't look as Paul had imagined. Like her jaw, her shoulders were broad and square, and except for lines temporarily stamped on her forehead when she finished a sentence with a question mark, her face was devoid of wrinkles. Her hair was black, not gray or white, her handshake beefy and strong, not boney and weak, her voice clear and resolute, not shaky and unclear and her eyes sparkled when she spoke. Not bad for 615 years old.

"Aren't you a sweet young man."

Paul looked at his own hands. Boney, wrinkled, spotted and old. Paul looked toward his feet, but couldn't see them as they were blocked by his vein covered, distended belly. He scratched the top of his hairless head and wiped sweat from creases that formed in his stubbled, weakened neck. Was she ancient and wise or simply deluded? Young man?

"One question. Ask it and I'll answer. If you have more than one question, you will need to return to the back of the line and when you reach the front again, you can ask your second question. We must treat everywhere fairly and given the many questioners, only one can be asked at a time. Your question please?"

Paul looked to his left and saw a line of hundreds snaking through small moguls of green grass interrupted by wooden

park benches and low hanging, puffy, white clouds. The line be-
gan ten feet from where Paul stood, behind a white line drawn
on the sidewalk that led to her throne, a black leather recliner,
with holes in the arm rests, ready for pop, beer or a glass full of
milk. On each side of the white line in the sidewalk separating
St. Peter from the masses, stood a pole holding a sign that read,
For the Privacy of Others, Remain Behind the Line Until Told
to Move Forward.

Paul didn't know he'd be limited to one question. He had so
many, questions about Bill, Frank and effort and contributions,
worthiness and relevance and wasn't prepared to ask just one, so
he took time to formulate the one question he was given and then
noticed she was becoming impatient with his silent stammering.
She began to clear her throat, brush non-existent strands of hair
from her smooth forehead, click her tongue in rhythm with Barry
Manilow music that fell from the sky and bob her head and raise
her eyebrows in anticipation of Paul's question. "Young man? A
question? Please. Others are waiting."

"Dad. Are you here?"

"Huh? Sorry, Aly. I must be drifting off."

"You said you had one question. Do you remember?"

"Sorry honey. I don't remember." Paul looked out the window
in the direction of Zion Lutheran. It was dark. He thought it had
been sunny the last time he looked from the window. He didn't
know how long he'd been tottering between sleep and wakeful-
ness, light and dark. Hours? Days? Tuesday? Wednesday?

"What day is it?" *"What day is it?"*

She smiled and tapped her staff to the ground. "So easy. It's Thursday. After standing in line waiting to talk to a 615 year old woman gatekeeper, most people ask questions with more depth, questions about life, death and the hereafter. But, the question is yours to ask, mine to answer. It's Thursday. Thank you for your interest."

"No wait. That was for Aly, not you. Can I have a do-over? I stood in line for what I think was hours, probably days. I'm not sure. It may have been light and then dark. I'm not sure. I've lost track of time. But, I didn't need you to determine what day it is. I could have looked at a calendar or my phone to determine what day it is. I didn't want to ask you what day it was. I didn't want to waste my opportunity. Can I ask another?"

Barry Manilow's voice disappeared and Paul heard a chorus of African American voices sing gospel. The song was familiar, but having missed church for months while battling cancer and waiting to die, Paul couldn't quite place it. His memory was foggy. He remembered the tune, not the words. The Old Rugged Cross? Onward Christian Soldiers? Proud Mary? He wasn't sure.

As Paul waited for another opportunity to uncover the secret of relative immortality, the choir spelled R-E-S-P-E-C-T and the very old woman in a young woman's clothes, the 615 year old who didn't look older than 59, the woman Paul believed had been given the power to determine the direction a questioner would travel, answered Paul's plea. "No. One question. That's it. Go to the back of the line if you have others."

Frustrated by the old woman's edict and his inability to name that tune, Paul lost his composure and as two very young men, one black, the other white, took him by the arm pits and began to lead him from the old woman's throne, he shouted, "What is that song?"

"Let's Get Together. Hayley Mills. From the Parent Trap. That's two. You've exceeded your limit. Be gone."

"The day? Thursday. Wanna watch the Twins? Probably seventh or eighth inning by now."

"No. Always another game."

Aly stood and took hold of a side-rail and squeezed, displacing blood in her hands, leaving her knuckles white. "You okay?"

"I'm fine for a dying man. Pain free, like a head in a bell jar. The drugs work. Can't feel much below the neck, which is probably good, given what I'd feel if I could feel."

Aly released the side-rail from captivity, brushed a lock from her forehead and asked, "Any reason why you're drifting in and out?"

"Probably, the meds, and the march toward oblivion. Sometimes it's hard to tell if I'm awake or asleep. I guess it's the price I pay for being pain free. The meds mask the pain, but they also cloud my reality and make it hard to stay awake. But, it's okay. As long as I can find what I need to enjoy life in short visits, it's okay. It's the price I need to pay, I guess. And when I'm gone, not gone-

gone, but asleep, I dream and the dreams are entertaining, maybe real, a preview of things to come. I'd rather talk to you, your mom and brother and sister, but when I can't, when the drugs pull me to sleep, I interact with Barry Manilow, a choir from Harlem and a 615 year old woman without wrinkles and perhaps the power to open the gate to Heaven, one question at a time."

"I never remember my dreams."

"I didn't until recently. I'm not sure why I remember them now. Maybe it's because they've become more vivid with drugs. Maybe it's because they're nearly as much a part of me now, as is my reality here with you. I've got a foot in and a foot out. The dreams may be my foot out. Not sure."

"Six-hundred-fifteen years old?"

Paul's eyelids dropped and a woman who stood in line with him, a woman who would ask a question immediately before Paul was given an opportunity to ask number three, answered the question Paul thought Alyson had asked. She was overweight, wore too much makeup and chewed on a toothpick. "Amazing. 615 years old. They examined her DNA, carbon dated her bones and asked her questions about the last 615 years, and concluded her claim is accurate. Born in 1400. Went to school with Joan of Arc, babysat Michelangelo's kids and convinced Columbus that he wouldn't fall from earth sailing west. Read Mac Beth on pages inked by Shakespeare the night before, sat at a piano with Vivaldi and brokered peace between England and the Colonies. One amazing woman."

"But how? How can she be 615?"

"High fat, low carb diet? God's benevolent touch? I don't know. No one does. Scientists are analyzing her blood, marrow, saliva, brain cells and urine. They're looking for answers. They hope to determine why she is ageless so they can make us all ageless." She flexed her bicep and asked, "Have you signed up?"

"For what? Signed up for what?" Paul hoped he had. He wasn't sure what he would have signed up for, but desperately wanted to know that he had. It seemed important. Life or death important.

"Agelessness. If you're not on the list, you won't benefit from the research. I'm on the list. I signed up the day, the hour, the minute, the second I was able to. She's 615 now. Who knows the limit. She looks so young, at 615? Maybe a thousand years, maybe more. I'm so glad I'm on the list. Are you?"

Paul checked his pockets. A receipt? A list that contained his name? His pockets were empty. "I don't think so. I don't remember."

"Too late for you." The large woman with an unprofessionally painted face, the woman on the list, the woman who attached her name to the list the moment she could, laughed, looked at the sidewalk, drew an imaginary line on the pavement with her eyes, stretched her fat arms and with palms extended in Paul's direction, told him to stay behind the line she drew with her imagination. Destined for death, precluded from relative immortality because he hadn't signed up, wasn't on the list, Paul heard the woman on the list whisper to the man who stood in front of her, "He's not on the list. Hope it's not catching."

Unwilling to cross the imaginary line, Paul stood still and watched those in line before him move forward in the direction of a 615 year old woman who sat in a black, leather recliner, creating a gap between those on the list and those not. It was Paul and then all of the others. He was excluded. Out. Not a member.

Alone, a football field away from those who neared the old/ young, 615 year old woman, Paul's chest began to hurt and his knees wobbled. As his knees buckled and he fell to the pavement, he drew in a sharp, deep breath, opened his eyes, fell to his soft bed with side-rails and saw Mary sitting on the chair adjacent to his bed, reading a book downloaded to her iPad.

After wiping sleep from his eyes and contemplating the old woman and immortality, Paul spoke to his wife who sat and read a book only feet away. "We're too old. We'll miss it."

"Miss what, Paul?"

"Immortality on earth. We're too old to live to be really old."

Mary put the iPad on her lap, smiled and asked the question Paul had requested she ask. "What do you mean?"

"Sooner or later, they'll figure it out. They'll learn how to slow down the aging process or how to clone us from our own cells so we can live over and over. But, we'll be dead before that happens, so we'll miss out."

"You'd choose immortality here on earth?"

"It'd be nice. I wouldn't be worried about day-after-tomorrow. If death is not part of the equation, there's nothing to worry about."

Mary lifted the iPad from her lap, stood, set the tablet on the table near the bed and hit some letters that appeared on the screen. After watching the pictures on the iPad screen change, she turned it toward Paul and said, "Nothing to worry about with immortality?"

Paul looked at the screen and read the words that appeared below a picture of Trump, who stood at a podium with clenched fists and a mouth opened wide and shaped like the opening of a raw sewage pipe. "Trump vows to ban Muslims from entering the United States, to keep America safe from evil. The Republican front runner spoke to a rabid crowd who cheered his vitriolic, mean-spirited campaign speech. Traditional Republicans maintain distance from the fiery candidate, however, afraid of antagonizing his zealous supporters, few speak out to disagree with his rhetoric."

Paul looked from the screen to Mary. He closed his eyes once, twice and the third time, they remained closed. A Muslim ban. Hateful speech. Popular? Stupid, yet beloved by many who want him to lead? *"Why Trump?"*

She removed a moisture laden Coors Light can from a hole in her throne's right arm, tipped it when it reached her lips and poured golden wet down her parched, 615 year old throat. She rested the can on her right thigh and then her left and when she returned it to the hole in the chair's arm, she looked at Paul with bright eyes on each side of her nose and sullen, hazy eyes imprinted by the wet can on her rather youthful, tight, thighs. "Unprecedented. In 615 years, I've never seen anything quite like Trump. Not smart. Not articulate. Not empathetic. Not experienced. Not honest. Not kind or persuasive. But, in spite of all that he doesn't have, he has a loyal following. Unprecedented."

Paul saw a black man and a white man emerge from behind the throne and walk his way. He recognized them. They'd been there before, in his bedroom, in his dream. They were there to take him away, to deposit him, either in a bed with side-rails or at the end of the line. Paul raised his palms in their direction, asking them to stop, while he pleaded with the ageless queen. "You haven't answered my question. I am entitled to an answer."

The very old woman in young skin looked at the approaching men and when she did, they stopped and waited their next command. "Sir, you are entitled to one question, but not an answer, especially when there isn't one. Why Trump? I have no idea. He has very little to give, so the answer is likely related to what others have not given. When people are filled with holes, they want them filled. Trump is the patch, the hot tar, the moist cement." She looked at the black man and the white man and, in unison, they marched to Paul and escorted him to the back of the line, to the bed with side-rails to keep the sick in bed.

"You okay Dad?"

Paul looked out the window. It was dark. Was it the same dark he saw when he talked to Mary. *Was it Mary? Or was it Aly? Paul?* Did he miss a day of sunshine or was the sunshine on its way? *Was Zion Lutheran still there?* Did it crumble under pressure from non-believers or those who believe too much? *Was there snow on the ground? Was the golf course open or were people skiing down the slopes at Buck Hill? August? January? Today? Tomorrow? Living? Dead?*

"It doesn't matter, Randy. It's all irrelevant. In the end, it doesn't matter."

Randy wiped sweat from Paul's forehead and walked to the window facing Paul's bed, which he opened wide with a twist of a handle. Paul felt a warm breeze liberated by the open window brush across his moist, uncovered face. *Summer. Golf, not downhill skiing.* "Irrelevant."

"Why irrelevant, Dad?"

"It could be January and I wouldn't know. People could be sliding over icy roads, and I wouldn't know. Zion could've been replaced by a Walmart, and I'd not know and if I did know, it wouldn't make any difference to me. If an earthquake separated California from the United States and it dropped into the Pacific, it wouldn't change what little life I have left. Death is liberating. Bullies can bully, young can die, preachers can condemn, cars can crash, countries can wage war and those in power can make catastrophic decisions, but nothing they do will change my life. I'm immune. I'm liberated. It's all irrelevant to me now."

"Is that a good thing, Dad?"

"It's not good or bad. It just is. While waiting to die, you're kinda dead. You don't change things and things don't change you.

388

Not influenced. Not influential. Maybe it means I'm accepting my fate and recognizing this is merely preparation, a place to plant seeds, a place to love, a place from which to matriculate. It's all been good, but what awaits is better. And I think I'm ready. I'm not 615 years old, but we've met and she approved."

Liberated, Paul smiled. Liberated, seeing more clearly than ever before, he spoke. "It's all good, Randy. All good."

Paul closed his eyes. While he could, he tried to open them, to see Randy, his room, his world, his family and his friends, but couldn't. And then, he stopped trying.

"Would you like to sit? Take my place on the throne?"

Paul sat on the leather recliner and as he did, the wrinkles in his skin disappeared. When he scratched the top of his head, his fingers wrestled thick, blonde hair and when he looked to his feet, his distended belly vanished and his feet tapped, keeping time with John Lennon, Frank Sinatra, Scott Joplin, Johnny Cash and Bobby Darin.

"You may ask as many questions as you like."

Trump? Doesn't matter. Why? Doesn't matter? How? Doesn't matter. None of it matters. "I have no questions."

"Would you like to fly?"

The side-rails, designed to keep the sick in bed, don't matter to the dead.

The cancer's onslaught was over. The pain was gone, his worries forgotten. He smiled. *"Yes, I'd like to fly."*

"Dad?"

"Paul?"

Paul didn't answer. As his family wept, as they held his cooling hand and remembered the nearly great man, in places unseen, he soared. And smiled.

The end.

about the author

Born in 1952, Kim Brandell was raised in Anoka, Minnesota and returned there after military service, college, law school and practice as a lawyer. A father of two and husband to one, Kim enjoys the characters in a book almost as much as litigants in a courtroom, opposing attorneys and judges, because unlike wonderful plaintiffs and defendants, competent and kind lawyers and the wise and warm men and women in black robes, he can tell fictional characters what to do and they do it.

From an author's perspective, the characters in a book are exactly as the author wants them to be. Life is simple in a book.

Hello

If you want to contact the author, Kim Brandell,
he'd be happy to hear from you.
Email him at kbrandellbooks@hotmail.com.